# 101 Skinny Meals In Minutes
## The Fast Weight Loss Cookbook

By Monique
Abercrombie-Wells

NMD Books
Simi Valley, CA

Library of Congress Cataloging-in-Publication
101 Skinny Meals In Minutes: The Fast Weight Loss Cookbook  by Monique
Abercrombie-Wells
ISBN:   978-1-936828-40-1 (Softcover)


First Edition January 2015

# Table of Contents

# Beef Dishes

## *Sloppy Joes*

4 teaspoons olive oil
2 onions, finely chopped
1 celery stalk, finely chopped
1/2 carrot, finely chopped
1/2 green bell pepper, seeded and finely chopped
1/2 teaspoon dried oregano leaves
1/2 teaspoon dried thyme leaves
1 pound lean ground beef
1 cup canned diced tomatoes
2 Tablespoons tomato paste
1 Tablespoon Worcestershire sauce
2 teaspoon red-wine vinegar
1/4 teaspoon hot red pepper sauce
Salt and pepper to taste
4 rolls or hamburger buns
4 unsweetened pickles (optional)

In a medium nonstick saucepan, heat the oil. Sauté the onions, celery, carrot and bell pepper until the onions are translucent, 10-12 minutes. Stir in the oregano and thyme, then add the beef and cook, breaking it apart with a wooden spoon, until no longer pink, 5-7 minutes.

In a small bowl, combine the tomatoes, tomato paste and 2 Tablespoons water, add to the beef mixture and cook 1 minute. Stir in the Worcestershire sauce, vinegar, pepper sauce, salt and pepper; bring to a boil. Reduce the heat and simmer, stirring occasionally, until the mixture thickens, about 10 minutes. Serve on the rolls with the pickles on the side.

Makes 4 servings, 9 points each. Serve these wonderfully messy joes on hard rolls with plenty of napkins on hand. If you like, you can also serve the meat over plain white rice.

# Mushroom Burgers

2 teaspoons olive oil
1/2 red or yellow bell pepper, seeded and finely chopped
1/2 onion, finely chopped
2 Tablespoons minced carrot
2 Tablespoons minced celery
2 garlic cloves, minced
2 cups finely chopped mushrooms
3/4 pound lean ground beef (10% or less fat)
1 Tablespoon steak sauce
Salt and freshly ground pepper, to taste

In a medium nonstick skillet, heat the oil. Sauté the bell pepper, onion, celery and garlic until the onion is translucent, 8 - 10 minutes. Add the mushrooms; sauté until the mushrooms brown and the liquid evaporates, about 8 minutes. Cool to room temperature.

Spray the broiler rack with nonstick cooking spray; preheat the broiler. In a medium bowl, combine the mushroom mixture, beef, steak sauce, salt and pepper. Form 4 hamburgers. Broil the burgers 3" - 4" from heat, 5-7 minutes on each side.

4 servings, 4 points each

# Ground Beef with Green Beans

1/4 lb. lean ground beef
1/2 cup chopped onions
2 cans cut green beans with liquid
8 oz. can tomato sauce
1/2 tsp. allspice
Salt and pepper to taste

Brown meat with onions. Drain well. Add green beans with liquid, tomato sauce and allspice. Simmer for about 20 minutes.

This is only 5 points for the entire recipe. You may add more beef and count the additonal points. One pound of 90% lean ground beef is 20 points, per my WW speaker.

# Breads and Muffins

## Breads

### Corn Bread

1 1/4 cups yellow cornmeal
3/4 cup all-purpose flour
4 teaspoon sugar
2 1/2 teaspoon baking powder
1/2 teaspoon salt
1 cup + 2 tablespoons low-fat buttermilk
1 egg

Preheat oven to 400 degrees. Spray an 8-inch square baking dish or 12-cup muffin tin with non-stick cooking spray. Combine cornmeal, flour, sugar, baking powder, and salt. In a small bowl, beat the buttermilk and egg.

Pour over the flour mixture; stir until blended. (do not overmix) Pour into pan or muffin tins. Bake until golden brown and a toothpick inserted in the center comes out clean.
(20-25 minutes)

12 servings , 2 points each

# Italian Calzones

1 bread dough -- frozen
1 pound extra lean ground beef -- round
1/2 cup mushrooms -- chopped
1/2 cup onion -- finely chopped
1/4 cup green bell pepper -- chopped
1/2 cup evaporated skim milk
3 tablespoons dry bread crumbs -- fine
1 1/2 teaspoons dried oregano
1/2 teaspoon crushed red pepper
1 teaspoon fennel seed -- crushed
3 cloves garlic -- minced
3/4 cup tomato sauce 1 teaspoon sugar
1/4 teaspoon salt
Vegetable cooking spray

Thaw bread dough.

Combine ground beef and next 9 ingredients in a large skillet; stir well. Cool over medium heat 10 minutes of until meat is browned, stirring to crumble meat. Add 3/4 cup tomato sauce, sugar, and salt; cook 6 minutes, stirring occasionally. (drain off excess grease when done).

Remove from heat; let mixture cool slightly. Divide dough into 8 equal portions. Working with 1 portion at a time (cover remaining portions to keep dough from drying out), roll each portion to 1/8-inch thickness. Place on a large baking dish coated with cooking spray, and pat each portion into a 6-inch circle with floured fingertips. Spoon

1/3 cup meat mixture onto half of each circle; moisten edges of dough with water. Fold dough over filling; press edges together with a fork to seal. Lightly coat with cooking spray.
4. Bake at 375 degrees for 20 minutes or until golden. Remove from oven, and lightly coat again with cooking spray. Serve warm.

8 servings, 5 points each

# "Red Lobster" Cheddar Biscuits

2 cups Bisquick, reduced-fat baking mix
3/4 cup lowfat buttermilk (1%fat)
1 cup shredded lowfat cheddar cheese
2 tbsp Fleischmann's Fat-Free Buttery Spread
1/4 tsp garlic powder
1/4 tsp dried parsley flakes, crushed fine

Preheat oven to 400 degrees. combine the baking mix, milk and cheddar cheese in a medium bowl. Mix by hand until well combined. Divide the dough into 12 equal portions (about 3 tbsp each) and spoon onto a lightly greased or nonstick cookie sheet. Flatten each biscuit a bit with your fingers.

Bake for 18 to 20 minutes or until the tops of the biscuits begin to brown. In a small bowl, combine the buttery spread with the garlic powder. Heat this mixture for 30 seconds in the microwave, then brush a light coating over the top of each biscuit. To make fine parsley flakes, as can be found on the original, simply crush the flakes between your thumb and forefinger.

12 servings, 2 points each

# _Muffins_

## _Banana Muffins_

3 large bananas, mashed
3/4 c sugar
1 egg
1 teaspoon baking soda
1 teaspoon baking powder
1/2 teaspoon salt
1-1/2 cup all purpose flour
1/3 cup applesauce (if you prefer you can use the cinnamon applesauce instead!)

Add sugar and slightly beaten egg to mashed bananas and mix well; add applesauce.

Make a well in the middle and add the dry ingredients, mix well but do not over mix. Bake at 375 for 20 minutes.

12 muffins, 3 points each

# Friendly Fiber Muffins

1 cup whole wheat flour
2 tsp. baking powder
1/2 tsp. salt
1 3/4 cups Kashi Good Friends cereal
3/4 cup skim milk, rice or soy milk
1/4 cup honey
2 egg whites
1/4 cup unsweetened applesauce
1 medium ripe banana, mashed non-stick cooking spray

Preheat oven to 400.

In a small bowl, stir together flour, baking powder and salt. Set aside.

In a large mixing bowl, combine Kashi Good Friends cereal and milk and let stand for 2-3 minutes. Add the egg whites and beat well. Stir in honey, applesauce and banana.

Add flour mixture and mix only until dry ingredients are moistened (over-mixing will produce rubbery muffins).

Fill sprayed muffin tins. Bake for 20-25 minutes or until lightly browned.

Makes 12 muffins, 1 point each

# *Cinnamon Bran Muffins*

2 cups Kelloggs All Bran Xtra Fiber Cereal
1 1/2 cup skim milk
1 1/4 cup flour
1/4 cup sugar
1 1/3 tbsp baking powder
1 tsp cinnamon
1/4 cup apple butter
1/3 cup egg substitute
1/4 cup raisins 1/4 cup walnuts

Combine cereal and milk in mid-size bowl. Sir to mix well and set aside for 15 minutes. Combine flour, sugar, baking powder, raisins and cinnamon in large bowl and stir to mix well. Add apple butter and egg substitute. Add cereal mixture to flour mixture and stir just until dry ingredients are moistened. Fold in walnuts.

Spray 12 regular-sized muffin tins with nonstick spray. Fill with batter. Bake at 350 degrees for 17 minutes or until toothpick inserted in the center comes out clean. Cool in pan for 5 minutes.

12 servings, 1 point each

# Carrot Banana Muffins

1 Cup brown sugar
1 Cup carrots
1 Cup bananas mashed
1/2 tsp cinnamon
1/2 cup applesauce
2 eggs
2 cups flour
1/2 tsp baking powder
1 tsp baking soda

Stir moist ingredients together, add dry ingredients. Spray muffin tin with cooking spray.. Bake 350 for 30 minutes)

12 servings, points each

# WW Bran Muffins

2 cups Whole Wheat Flour
3 cups White Flour
5 tsp. Baking Soda
1 tsp. salt
1 1/2 cups Brown sugar
3 Cups Natural Bran
3 cups All Bran
2 cups Raisins
2 eggs & 2 egg whites
1 cup apple sauce
1/4 cup molasses
1 quart 1% buttermilk
1 1/2 cups water

Set oven to 375 degrees.

Mix all dry ingredients in "large" mixing bowl. Beat eggs &
liquids all together in separate bowl. Make a "well" in middle of
dry stuff. Add liquids to "well" & mix thoroughly. Let batter sit for
5 minutes - then fill muffin tins 2/3 full.

Bake for 17-20 minutes.

Freeze & use as needed.

5 dozen muffins, 1 point each

# Pumpkin-Bran Muffins

Nonstick Cooking Spray
2 cups All-Bran or Fiber One cereal
1 cup skim milk
3/4 cup pumpkin
2 teaspoon pumpkin pie spice
1 egg
1/2 cup brown sugar
1 1/4 cup flour
1 tablespoon baking powder
1 teaspoon salt

Mix together and let rest for 5 minutes: cereal and milk. Add pumpkin, egg, pumpkin pie spice and brown sugar.

Mix together flour, salt, baking powder and add to pumpkin mixture. Spray 12 regular-sized muffin tins with nonstick spray. Bake at 350 degrees for 15-17 minutes or until toothpick inserted in the center comes out clean.

Cool in pan for 5 minutes.

12 servings, 1 point each

# Casseroles

## *Broccoli & Chicken Casserole*

3 cups noodles -- "No Yolk"
2 1/2 cups ground chicken, cooked
1/2 cup onions, chopped
3 1/4 cups frozen broccoli flowerets, thawed
1 (10 3/4 oz.) can Cream of Celery, lowfat condensed
1/2 cup skim milk
1/2 cup Swiss cheese, low-fat shredded
1 teaspoon basil
2 teaspoons salt
1/4 teaspoon black pepper

Preheat oven at 350 degrees. Prepare a 2 1/2-quart casserole dish with cooking spray; set aside. Cook noodles according to package directions. Drain. Cook ground chicken rinsing under very hot water to remove any excess fat. In a mixing bowl, combine noodles, chicken, onions, and broccoli. In another mixing bowl, combine soup, milk, cheese, basil, salt, and pepper. Stir in noodle mixture. Pour entire mixture into prepared dish. Bake, covered for 40 minutes.

7 points

# Cabbage Roll Casserole

1 pound extra lean ground beef, cooked and drained
1 head cabbage, chopped
1 can tomato soup
1 medium onion, chopped
1 cup rice, cooked and drained
3 tablespoons Worcestershire sauce
1 teaspoon salt
1 teaspoon pepper

Brown ground beef with chopped onions and Worcestershire sauce. Place half the chopped cabbage on bottom of baking pan. Top with half the cooked beef mixture.

Spread half of the rice over the meat mixture. (You may add rice directly to the beef mixture and spread over the cabbage.) Repeat with a layer of cabbage and another layer of the meat mixture. Mix the tomato soup with a can of water. Pour this over casserole. Cover with aluminum foil and bake at 350 degrees for 1 hours.

6 servings, 7 points each

# Baked Cauliflower Casserole

4 cups, cauliflower florets, blanched
1/2 c. tomato sauce
1 1/2 oz. mozzarella cheese, shredded
2 Tablespoons grated Parmesan cheese

Preheat oven to 375 degrees. Spray 9 inch glass pie pan with nonstick cooking spray. Arrange cauliflower in pie plate and spoon tomato sauce over cauliflower.

In small mixing bowl, combine cheeses; sprinkle over tomato sauce.

Bake until cauliflower is thouroughly heated, about 15 minutes.

Makes 4 servings, 1 point each

Approximate total time: 30 minutes (including baking time)


# Chicken Casserole

1 large canned chicken
1 bag egg noodles, yolk-free -- medium
4 ounces chopped broccoli, frozen -- thawed slightly
4 ounces peas -- small
1 carrot -- chopped
1 can cream of celery soup, condensed
1 can cream of chicken soup (98 % fat free)

Boil noodles according to directions. Drain and place back into pot. Mix together all ingredients and place into a 13x9 pan. Bake for 30 minutes, covered.

6 servings, 4 points each

# Cheesy Eggplant Casserole

1 1/3 cups onion, chopped
2 cloves garlic
11 ounces whole tomatoes, canned
2 tablespoons tomato paste
3/4 cup fat-free mozzarella cheese
3/4 cup cottage cheese, lowfat
2 tablespoons Parmesan cheese, grated
3/4 pound eggplant, slices 1/2" thick
1 tablespoon parsley
3/4 teaspoon oregano, ground
1/3 teaspoon basil, ground

Coat a large skillet with nonstick cooking spray. Add the onion and garlic to the skillet and sauté over low heat until onion is tender, about 6 minutes. Stir in drained whole tomatoes, tomato paste, parsley, oregano, basil and salt and pepper to taste. Bring mixture to a boil, reduce heat and let simmer, uncovered, for 40-50 minutes, stirring occasionally.

Arrange eggplant slices on a steamer rack. Place in a large pot to which 1inch of water has been added, and steam for about 5 minutes until eggplant is tender. Do not overcook. Combine the mozzarella and cottage cheeses together and set aside. Coat a 13"x9" baking pan with nonstick cooking spray and place a layer of eggplant in the pan. Top eggplant with some of the sauce mixture and some of the cheese mixture and sprinkle with Parmesan cheese. Repeat the steps in layers until all the ingredients are used. Bake at 350 for 30-35 minutes and serve hot.

4 Servings, 3 points each

# Easy Corn Casserole

1/4 cup egg beaters® 99% egg substitute
1/4 cup margarine, melted
1 corn, whole kernel, canned (8.75 oz) drained
01corn, cream-style, (8.85 oz)
01pkg. corn muffin mix, (8.5 oz)
01carton sour cream, reduced fat, (8oz) Cooking spray

Preheat oven to 350. Combine first 6 ingredients in a med. bowl, stir well. Pour into an

8-inch square baking dish sprayed with cooking spray. Bake at 350 for 45 minutes or until set.

8 servings, 3 points each

# Mac N Cheese

4 cups hot cooked elbow macaroni(about 8 oz uncooked),
cooked with salt or fat
2 cups (8 ozs) shredded reduced-fat sharp cheddar cheese
1 cup 1% low fat cottage cheese
 3/4 cup ff sour cream
1/2 cup skim milk
2 Tblsp grated fresh onion
1 1/2 tsps reduce-calorie stick margarine, melted
1/2 tsp salt
1/4 tsp pepper
1 large egg, lightly beaten cooking spray
1/4 cup fresh or dry bread crumbs
1 Tblsp reduced-calorie stick margarine, melted
1/4 tsp paprika

Preheat oven to 350.

Combine first 10 ingredients, stir well. Spoon into a shallow 2-qt
casserole coated with cooking spray.

Combine breadcrumbs, 1 tbsp margarine, and paprika; stir well.
Sprinkle breadcrumb mixture over casserole. Cover and bake
45 min. Uncover and bake 5 more minutes until breadcrumbs
are lightly brown.

6 cups=8 pts

# Layered Tortilla Bake

1 pound lean ground beef
1 can dark red kidney beans, drained & rinsed
1 can (28 oz) tomato, chopped
1 can (4 oz) chopped green chilies (mild)
1 pkg. (1.25 oz) McCormick's 30% less sodium Taco Seasoning
1 pkg. (10 oz) corn tortillas (12, 6-inch tortillas)
1 Cup (4 oz) shredded low fat cheddar cheese

Preheat oven to 350 degrees. Brown ground beef in large
nonstick skillet; drain well. Mix in beans, tomatoes, chilies and
taco seasoning mix. Reduce heat; simmer 5 min.
Spray 9 x 13 " baking dish with nonstick cooking spray.

Cut tortillas in half place half of them in bottom of baking dish,
overlapping. Spoon half of beef mixture evenly over tortillas.
Cover with remaining tortillas and then remaining beef mixture.
Top with cheese. Cover; bake 25 minutes.

8 servings, 5 points each

# Pizza Casserole

1 lb. lean ground beef
1/2 cup green peppers
1 cup onion
15 ounces tomato sauce
1 teaspoon garlic powder
1/2 teaspoon oregano
1/2 teaspoon onion salt
1/4 teaspoon pepper
4 oz. grated cheddar cheese
2 ounces non-fat Parmesan cheese
1 cup canned mushrooms
4 1/2 oz. egg noodles, uncooked

Brown ground beef, green pepper, and onion. Add tomato sauce, garlic powder, oregano, onion salt and pepper and simmer for 15 min. Cook noodles. Pour sauce over noodles and sprinkle with cheddar cheese and Parmesan cheese. Top with mushrooms. Cover with foil. Bake 400 degrees for 10 minutes. Freezes well.

6 servings, 7 points each

# Quick Tuna Casserole

5 ounces noodles, egg, cooked
3 cups boiling water
1 can cream of mushroom soup (98 % fat free)
1/3 cup skim milk
1 can tuna in water, canned (6.5 ounce)
1 cup peas, canned
1 cup bread crumbs

Preheat oven to 350. Cook noodles in boiling water for 2 minutes. Remove from heat, cover and let stand for 10 minutes. Meanwhile, in a medium bowl mix together soup, milk, tuna and peas. Rinse noodles and drain well. Add to the tuna mixture. Pour into an

8" x 8" spray baking dish. Sprinkle with breadcrumbs. Spray top with "I Can't Believe its not Butter" if desired. Bake 30 minutes. 6 servings, 4 points each

# Nacho Casserole

1 c. salsa
4 oz canned chiles
1/4 t. cumin
1/2 c. plain yogurt
1/4 c. water
1 lb hamburger
1/2 c. onion
1 c. refried beans
1 c. reduced fat shredded cheddar
4 c. corn flakes

Mix salsa and chillis, set aside. Brown hamburger and onions - add cumin, beans, yogurt, 1/2 cheese, 1/2 salsa and water.

Place 2 c. cornflakes in 9 x 13 pan. Spoon with meat mix and rest of salsa. Add remaining cornflakes on top.

Bake at 35 for 35 min. - top with remaining cheese and bake 5 minutes more.

6 servings, 5 points each


# Potato Casserole

32 ounces southern style hashbrowns thawed
8 ounces fat free sour cream
1 10 ounce can reduced fat cream of chicken soup
1 Cup evaporated skim milk
4 ounces reduced fat cheese

Combine all ingredients and place in 9x13 baking dish. Bake 350 degrees for 1 hour. 8 servings, 3 points each

# Reuben Casserole

1/4 c. fat free mayonnaise
1/4 c. fat free 1000 island dressing
2 c. sauerkraut - drained
1 pkg sliced 90% lean corned beef 2.5 oz pkg
3/4 c. WW reduced fat shredded Swiss cheese
1 c. fresh tomato - sliced
2 slices rye bread, low calorie - cut into pieces

Preheat oven to 350 degrees.

In a small bowl, combine mayonnaise and thousand island dressing. Layering in 8 x8" baking dish, place sauerkraut on bottom, corned beef, dressing mixture, Swiss cheese and tomatoes.

In a non stick pan sprayed with butter flavored spray, lightly sauté bread. Sprinkle on top of tomatoes.

Bake 20 minutes. 2 servings, 2 points each


# Spinach Casserole

2 packages spinach -- chopped
2 cups cottage cheese, lowfat
1/2 cup Egg Beaters® 99% egg substitute
1/2 cup Parmesan cheese (fat free) Paprika - to taste

Cook spinach until heated through. Drain very thoroughly, squeeze out the excess water. Combine the cottage cheese, egg substitute, and parmesan cheese in bowl. Mix in spinach. Pour into a 9 inch pie pan or into 6 individual baking dishes which have been sprayed with nonstick spray. Sprinkle casserole with a little parmesan and paprika.

Bake at 375* for 25 to 30 minutes, or until firm and lightly browned at the edges. 6 servings, 2 points each

# Vegetable Casserole

2 cans French Style green beans, drained
1 can corn, drained
1 can sliced water chestnuts, drained and diced
1 can Fat Free Cream of Celery soup
1 cup Fat Free or Lite sour cream
1 cup grated cheddar cheese

Combine green beans, corn, water chestnuts. Place into casserole dish. Mix together soup, sour cream and cheese and add to vegetables. Microwave until heated thoroughly.

Points per serving depends on type of sour cream and cheese that you choose.

# Desserts

## *Angel Food Cherry Cake*

1 package angel food cake mix
1 can light cherry pie filling

Preheat oven to 350 degrees. Mix both ingredients together and pour into a 9 x 13 baking dish. Bake for about 15 to 20 minutes. Makes 12 servings, 3 points each


## *Apple Crisp*

4 medium apples, cored, sliced and peeled
1/2 teaspoon cinnamon
3 tablespoons flour
1 tablespoon margarine
1/2 cup apple juice, unsweetened; concentrate

<u>Crispy Oat Topping</u>

1/3 cup flour
1/2 cup rolled oats
3 tablespoons margarine 1/4 teaspoon cinnamon

Preheat oven to 350°F. Spray a 9 x 9 x 2-inch baking dish with oil. In a large bowl, stir together all ingredients except topping. Pour mixture into prepared dish and crumble topping over. Bake 1 hour or until topping is crisp looking and slightly golden. Remove dish from oven and place on a wire rack to cool. Serve warm or cold. Store uncovered cooled crisp in refrigerator. Freeze in portions. In a medium-sized bowl, mix all ingredients with a fork.

Spoon topping over any pie or fruit mixture. 8 servings, 3 points each.

# Caramel-Apple Crisps

6 (4-inch) fat-free caramel-flavored popcorn cakes
1 medium apple, cored and thinly sliced (recommended using either a Golden Delicious or a Red Delicious apple)
1 1/2 tablespoons fat-free caramel-flavored sundae syrup
1 tablespoon brown sugar
1/2 teaspoon ground cinnamon

Place popcorn cakes on a baking sheet. Top evenly with sliced apple; drizzle caramel syrup evenly over apple.

Combine brown sugar and cinnamon; sprinkle evenly over each serving. Broil 3 minutes. Serve immediately.

6 servings, 2 points each


# Chocolate Peanut Butter Pie

4 tbsp. peanut butter
1 tbsp. honey
1 1/2 c. rice krispies
1 package chocolate sugar free pudding
2 c. skim milk
4 tbsp. Light cool whip

In a small bowl, combine peanut butter and honey. Microwave on high 20 seconds. Stir in cereal. Press into 9' pie plate. Chill.

Prepare pudding with skim milk (following package directions. Pour over piecrust. Chill.

Garnish with whipped topping. 8 servings, 2 points each

# Fluffy Pineapple Dessert

1 box of sugar free white chocolate instant pudding
1 middle sized can of crushed pineapple with juice
1 carton fat free cool whip medium size

Mix these 3 ingredients together and it is wonderful!
4 pts per serving.

# Jell-O

1 package cherry Jell-O (or any flavor you prefer)
1/2 cup applesauce
1 can (12 oz) ginger ale
1 20 oz can crushed pineapple(drained)

Heat applesauce and mix in Jell-O. Remove from heat and add ginger ale and pineapple. Stir completely. Pour into individual containers and chill until firm. Makes 6 servings-1 pt each.

# Lemon-Raspberry Cloud

1/4 c. lemon juice
2 Tablespoons thawed frozen concentrated orange juice
1 Tablespoon granulated sugar
1/2 tsp. grated lemon peel
1 tsp. unflavored gelatin
1/2 c. Kool Whip
3 egg whites
1/4 tsp. cream of tartar
1/2 c. raspberries

In small nonstick saucepan, combine lemon juice, 1/4 c. water, the o.j., sugar and lemon peel; sprinkle gelatin over juice mixture and let stand 1 minute to soften. Stir mixture to combine; cook over low heat, stirring frequently until gelatin is dissolved, 1 to 2 minutes.

Transfer mixture to large mixing bowl; stir in whipped topping and set aside.

Using mixer on high speed, in large mixing bowl, beat egg whites until frothy; add cream of tartar and continue beating until whites are stiff but not dry. Gently fold egg whites into gelatin mixture utnil mixture is thoroughly combined.

Into each of 4 6 oz. dessert dishes, put 1/4 of gleatin mixture. Cover and refrigerate until firm, at least 1 hour (when gelatin mixture is chilled, it will form 2 layers.) Garnish each portion with 2 Tablespoons of raspberries.

Makes 4 servings, 1 point each

# Mounds Pudding

1 (4-serving size) Jell-O sugar-free instant white chocolate pudding mix 2/3 cup Carnation Nonfat Dry Milk powder
1 cup Water
3/4 Cup Yoplait plain fat -free yogurt 3/4 cup Cool Whip Free (I use Lite)
1 1/2 teaspoons Coconut extract
2 tablespoons (1/2 oz) Mini Chocolate Chips
2 tablespoons Hershey's Lite Chocolate Syrup
2 tablespoons Flaked Coconut

In a large bowl, combine dry pudding mix, dry milk powder, water and yogurt. Mix well using a wire whisk. Do not over mix.

Blend in Cool Whip Free (Lite) and coconut extract. Stir in chocolate chips. Evenly spoon mixture into 6 dessert dishes. Top each with 1 teaspoon chocolate syrup and 1 teaspoon coconut. Refrigerate for at least 15 minutes.

6 servings, 3 points each

# Low Fat Cake

## Cake

1 yellow cake mix
1 small can mandarin oranges with juice
3/4 c. applesauce
8 egg whites

Mix well. Spray and flour 9 x 13 pan. Bake 350 degrees for 30 minutes

## Topping

1 8 oz Cool-Whip fat free
1 20 oz crushed pineapple
1 small sugar free vanilla instant pudding

Mix pineapple juice with dry pudding, mix well and fold in Cool-Whip. Spread on cake

12 servings - 2 points each

# Chocolate Cream Pie

Low fat graham cracker pie crust

1 pkg fat free sugar free instant chocolate pudding mix 2 cups skim milk

Whip up to pudding; add fat free cool whip, 8 oz or less. Dump into crust; let set for 4 hours in fridge before serving

6 servings, 4 points each

# Creamy Chocolate Cheese Pie

Reduced fat Graham Cracker crust
Jell-O instant sugar free chocolate pudding (4 serving size)
8oz Fat Free Cream Cheese
1 cup Fat Free Yogurt
2 cups Cool Whip Free (thawed)

Mix together the cream cheese and yogurt until smooth. Add pudding mix and blend well. Fold in 1 cup of Cool Whip Free. Pour into pie shell. Chill until set (about 30 minutes).

Frost with remaining Cool Whip Free. Serves 8.

4 servings, 4 points each

# Chocolate Zucchini Cake

1 pkg Sweet Rewards Chocolate cake mix
1 c. applesauce unsweetened
3 eggs
2 c. shredded zucchini

Pour into 9 x 13 pan

Bake 350 degrees vor 35-40 minutes

12 servings. 3.5 points each

# *Pumpkin Cheesecake*

24 oz non-fat cream cheese (room temperature)
3/4 c. pumpkin
1/2 c. sugar
1 t. vanilla

Mix above ingredients on high speed then add: 3/4 c. egg substitute, 1/2 t. cinnamon, 1/4 t. cloves; blend well.

Spray 9" pie plate, Sprinkle with 2 T. graham cracker crumbs.

Bake 45 minutes at 325 degrees until set but not firm. Serve with Cool whip 8 servings, 3 points each

# Wildberry Cheesecake

Crust

Vegetable cooking spray
1 1/2 cups graham cracker crumbs
1/4 cup apple juice with vitamin C

Filling

2 Tbsp. unflavored gelatin 1/2 cup water
2 cups 1% fat cottage cheese
1 cup nonfat ricotta cheese
1 package (8-oz.) lite cream cheese
1/4 cup sugar
1 Tbsp. vanilla extract
1/2 cup mixed fruit puree

For crust: Preheat oven to 350 degrees F. Spray 9" spring form pan with cooking spray and set aside. In medium bowl, stir crumbs and apple juice until well combined. With back of spoon press crumb mixture evenly into prepared pan. Bake 5 minutes. Cool.

For filling: In small saucepan sprinkle gelatin over water; let stand 5 minutes to soften. Cook over low heat until dissolved, stirring often. Set aside. In food processor or blender process gelatin mixture and next 5 ingredients until smooth. Stir in fruit puree. Pour into prepared crust. Refrigerate at least 2 hours before serving.

10 servings, ___ points each Nutrition per serving: 180 calories and 2 grams of fat.

# Pumpkin Pudding

1-16 oz can of pumpkin
1 package of fat free, sugar free, vanilla or butterscotch pudding
Fat free Cool Whip (about 2 cups or more-depending on how much you want)

Mix pumpkin and pudding. Add cool whip. Refrigerate.

3 points

# Strawberry Pie

Combine 1 small pkg of sugar free vanilla cook and serve pudding with 2 cups of water and bring to a boil.

Stir in 1 small pkg sugar free strawberry Jell-O till dissolved.

Spread 4 cups of strawberries in a pie plate and pour the pudding/Jell-O mixture over them. Chill.

6 servings, 1 point each

# Weight Watcher Chocolate, Chocolate Brownie

1 can black beans drained and dried good.
1 cup water.
1 box Betty Crocker sweet reward mix and your blender.
Cupcake liners

Preheat oven to 350

After draining and drying beans put them in the blender w/ the 1 cup of water. Blend until liquidy.

in a medium mixing bowl mix the whole box of sweet reword w/ the bean mix. Mix until well blended.

Fill the cup cake cup 2/3 full. Put on a baking sheet and bake according to the brownie directions.

Make about 18 brownies, 2 points each

Tip: Freeze the brownie and eat them cold or just to keep them longer.

# Frozen Butterfinger Pie

40 Chocolate graham crackers (10 full sheets)
1 1/2 Tbsp butter or stick margarine, melted
1 large egg white cooking spray
2 cups vanilla fat-free frozen yogurt
3 Tbsp light-colored corn syrup
3 Tbsp creamy peanut butter
1 Tbsp fat-free milk
1 (2.1 ounce) chocolate-covered crispy peanut-buttery candy bar, such as Butterfinger, chopped.

Preheat oven to 350 degrees. Place graham crackers in a food processor: pulse until crumbly.

Add butter and egg white: pulse until moist. Press crumb mixture into a 9-inch pie plate coated with cooking spray. Bake at 350 for 8 minutes; cool on a wire rack 15 minutes. Freeze 15 minutes.

Remove yogurt from freezer, and let stand at room temperature for 15 minutes to soften. Spoon half of yogurt into prepared crust. Combine the corn syrup, peanut butter, and milk in a small bowl, stirring until smooth. Drizzle half of the peanut butter mixture over the yogurt in crust. Sprinkle with half of chopped candy bar. Repeat the procedure with remaining yogurt, peanut butter mixture, and candy bar. Cover with plastic wrap, and freeze for 3 hours or until firm.

Makes 9 servings, 5.5 points each (but worth saving points for)

# Caramel-Apple Salad

4 medium apples -- peeled, cored, diced
1 can crushed pineapple in light syrup -- (20 oz) drained
1 package butterscotch pudding (Jell-O sugar free) -- 1 oz. box
1 tub Cool Whip Lite® -- (8 oz)

Mix all ingredients thoroughly, refrigerate. Serving size 1/2 cup.
2 Points

# Baked Apples

4 Granny Smith apples or Rome apples, any hard apple <u>Syrup</u>

Boil Together:
1/4 cup plus 2 tablespoons water
2 tablespoons orange juice
3 tablespoons brown sugar
2 tablespoons granulated sugar
1 pinch cinnamon
1 teaspoon lemon juice
2 teaspoons lemon zest
1/8 teaspoon salt
1 tablespoon brown sugar (optional) -- to top

Heat oven to 350ºF. Mix together syrup ingredients and bring to
a boil. Peel the apples, removing only about the top two inches.
Core the apples and place them upright in a baking dish. Pour
the syrup over and into the apples. Cover with foil and bake for
30 minutes. A fork will glide through the apple when done.
Sprinkle tops with a little extra brown sugar and broil for 3
minutes. Serve warm with ice cream, whipped cream, crème
fraîche or plain cream.

NOTE : Simple and perfect without much fuss: one of the all-
time great desserts.

4 servings, 2 points each

# Watermelon Sorbet

4 cups watermelon chunks
1/4 cup superfine sugar
2 tablespoons lime juice

In a processor or blender, combine watermelon, sugar and lime juice; puree until smooth. Pour mixture into freezer safe container for 4-6 hours until set like gelatin. Spoon evenly into 4 desert dishes.

4 servings, 2 points each

# Egg Dishes

## *Breakfast Frittata*

2 teaspoons vegetable oil, divided
2 small red or green bell peppers, cut into strips (about 1 1/2 cups)
1/2 cup red onion strips
1/3 cup sliced green onion
6 small red-skinned potatoes, thinly sliced (about 1 1/2 cups)
4 egg whites
2 tablespoons skim milk
1/4 teaspoon salt

Preheat the broiler. In a 9-or 10-inch nonstick, heatproof skillet, heat 1 teaspoon of oil over medium heat. Add bell peppers and red and green onions; sauté until vegetables begin to soften, about 4 minutes. Add potatoes; cook until lightly browned, about 4 minutes. In a medium bowl, whisk together egg whites, egg, milk, and salt.

Add remaining oil to skillet and reduce heat to low. Pour in egg mixture. Cover and cook until eggs are set around edges but center is still loose, about 8 minutes. Using a rubber spatula, gently loosen egg mixture from sides of pan. Place skillet on the broiler rack; broil 4 inches from heat until Frittata is golden brown, about 1 minute. Gently slide Frittata onto a plate; cut into wedges. Tips: Loosen the Frittata from the pan by slipping a rubber spatula between the Frittata and skillet. Slide the Frittata carefully, in one piece, onto a plate.

3 points

# WW Quiche

16 ounces cottage cheese, lowfat
3 eggs
2 ounces Swiss cheese
1 box spinach -- drained & chopped
1 medium onion -- chopped
1 teaspoon oregano

Mix ingredients together. Lightly grease a 9" pie plate and pour in mixture. Bake at 350 degrees for 1 hour. You may use Egg Beaters if you like, enough for 3 eggs.

6 servings, 3 points each

# Easy Garden Bake (Crustless Quiche)

1 cup chopped zucchini
1 large tomato, chopped (1 cup)
1 medium onion, chopped (1 cup)
1/3 cup grated Parmesan cheese
1/2 cup Bisquick® Reduced fat baking mix
1 cup fat-free (skim) milk
1/2 cup fat-free cholesterol-free egg substitute
1/2 teaspoon salt
1/8 teaspoon pepper

Heat oven to 400°. Grease 9-inch pie plate. Layer zucchini, tomato, onion and cheese in pie plate. Stir remaining ingredients until blended. Pour into pie plate.

Bake about 35 minutes or until knife inserted in center comes out clean. Cool 5 minutes.

High Altitude (3500-6500 ft): Increase baking mix to 3/4 cup and bake time to 35-40 min.

1 serving, 2 points

# Fish and Seafood

## *Oven "Fried" Scallops*

15 oz. sea scallops, cut into quarters
3 Tablespoons low fat buttermilk
1/3 c. plus 2 tsps. seasoned dried bread crumbs
1/2 tsp. ground thyme

Preheat oven to 500 degrees. Spray baking sheet with nonstick cooking spray and set aside.

In med. mixing bowl, combine scallops and buttermilk, turning to coat; let stand at room temperature for 15 minutes to marinate.

In small mixing bowl, combine bread crumbs and thyme. Dredge each scallop in bread crumb mixture coating both sides, and arrange scallops on prepared baking sheet.

Bake, carefully turning scallops over until browned on all sides, about 5 minutes.

Makes 4 servings, 3 points each

Approximate total time: 10 minutes

# Oven Baked Fish and Chips

3 lb. baking Potatoes
3 Tbsp. Olive Oil divided
1/2 tsp. salt
1.4 tsp. pepper
1 tsp. chopped fresh rosemary (or 1/4 tsp. dried)
011.2 lb. white-fleshed fish fillets
011/4 cups all-purpose flour
2 egg whites or equivalent egg substitute to equal 1 egg
3/4 cup dry bread crumbs
3/4 cup Cornflake crumbs

Peel or scrub potatoes and cut into thick French-fry shapes. Pat dry and toss with 1 Tbsp. oil, salt, pepper and rosemary. Arrange in single layer on non-stick baking sheet or baking pan lined with parchment paper. Bake in preheated 425 degree oven for 40 minutes.

Meanwhile, cut fish into 6 serving-sized pieces. Pat dry. Place flour in shallow dish. Beat egg whites or put substitute in another shallow dish and combine breadcrumbs and Cornflake crumbs in third dish.

Dust each piece of fish with flour. Dip into egg whites and allow excess to run off. Dip into crumb mixture and pat crumbs in firmly.

While potatoes are cooking, brush second baking sheet with 1 tbsp. oil or line with parchment paper. Arrange fish in single layer on baking sheet and drizzle with remaining 1 Tbsp. oil. Put second baking sheet with fish in oven when potatoes have cooked for 40 minutes. Bake fish for 5 minutes, turn carefully and bake for 5 minutes or until fish is cooked through.

6 servings, 9 points each

# Mexican Dishes

## *Baked Chimichangas*

8 oz. cooked chicken (1-1/2 cups)
1 (8oz) jar salsa
01(16oz) can fat-free refried beans
01(4-1/2oz) can diced green chili peppers, drained
013 tablespoon thinly sliced green onions
4 oz reduced fat Monterey Jack or cheddar cheese, shredded (1 cup)
8 (8-9 inch) flour tortillas
Fat-free sour cream (optional)
Salsa (optional)
Thinly sliced green onion (optional)

Using 2 forks shred cooked poultry, pork, or beef. In a large skillet combine poultry or meat, the salsa, beans, chili peppers, and the green onions. Cook and stir over medium heat until heated through. Stir in cheese.

Meanwhile, wrap tortillas in foil warm in a 350 degrees oven for 10 minutes. For each chimichanga, spoon about 1/2-cup meat mixture on a tortilla, near one edge. Fold in sides; roll up. 3. Place in a 13 x 9 x 2-inch baking pan.

Bake, uncovered, in a 350-degree oven for 15 to 20 minutes or until heated through and tortillas are crisp and brown. If desired, serve with sour cream, additional salsa, and/or green onion.

8 servings, 7 points each

# Vegetable Quesadillas

1/4 c. seeded and diced tomato
1/4 c. diced yellow pepper
1/4 c. diced red pepper
2 Tablespoons chopped scallion (green onion)
1 tsp. seeded and chopped hot chili pepper
1 tsp. copped fresh cilantro or Italian parsley
2 flour tortillas (reduced- fat, 98% fat free)
1 1/2 Oz. reduced-fat Monterey Jack cheese, shredded
1 tsp. vegetable oil.

In small mixing bowl, combine tomato, bell peppers, scallions, chili pepper, and cilantro; set aside.

In 10 inch nonstick skillet, cook 1 tortilla over medium heat until flexible, about 1 minute on each side. Transfer tortilla to a plate.

Top half of tortilla with half of the cheese and then with half of the vegetable mixture; fold tortilla in half to cover filling. Repeat procedure with remaining tortilla, cheese and vegetable mixture.

In same skillet heat oil; add tortillas and cook until cheese is melted, 1 to 2 minutes on each side. Cut each tortilla in half.

Makes 2 servings, 2.5 points each. Approximate total time: 15 minutes

# Low-fat Layered Bean Dip

3 1/2 cups refried beans, fat free
2 cups sour cream, reduced fat
2 cups salsa
1 cup fat-free cheddar cheese

Place in a shallow bowl / pie plate about 2" deep the refried beans, then the sour cream, then the salsa, and top it off with the cheedar cheese. Keep refrigerater till ready to serve.

16 ( approx 1/2 cup) servings., 2 points each

# Cheese Crisp

1 flour tortilla (6 in. diameter)
1/4 c. chopped drained canned mild chili or jalapeno pepper
1 1/2 oz. reduced-fat Colby or Cheddar cheese, shredded
(optional- 1 Tablespoon sour cream- pts. don't include it)

Preheat broiler. Arrange tortilla directly on oven rack, 6 inches from heat source, and broil until lightly toasted, 1 to 2 minutes on each side.

Transfer tortilla to baking sheet; top with pepper and sprinkle with cheese. Broil until cheese is melted, 1 to 2 minutes.

To serve, arrange tortilla on serving plate and top with sour cream (optional).

Makes 1 serving, 2 points each

Approximate total time: 10 minutes

# Mexican Steak Stir-Fry

3/4 pound beef boneless sirloin, cut into 1 x 1/2 inch pieces 1
medium onion, chopped (1/2 cup)
1 small green bell pepper, chopped (1/2 cup)
1 small frozen whole kernel corn 1/2 cup salsa
1 medium zucchini, sliced (2 cups)
1 can (16 oz) pinto beans, rinsed and drained
1 can (14.5 oz) no-salt-added whole tomatoes, undrained.

Spray 12" nonstick skillet with nonstick cooking spray; heat over
medium-high heat.

Cook beef, onion and bell pepper in skillet 4 to 5 minutes,
stirring frequently, until beef is no longer pink.

Stir in remaining ingredients, breaking up tomatoes. Cook about
5 minutes, stirring occasionally until zucchini is tender and
mixture is hot.

4 points per serving

# Pasta

## *Super-easy Chicken Manicotti*

1 jar (26 to3 0oz) spaghetti sauce
1 teaspoon garlic salt
1 1/2 pounds chicken breast strips
14 uncooked manicotti shells (8oz)
2 cups shredded mozzarella cheese
Chopped fresh basil, if desired

Heat oven to 350. Spread about 1/3 of the spaghetti sauce in ungreased 9x13x2 pan.

Sprinkle garlic salt on chicken. Insert chicken into uncooked shell, stuffing from each end of shell to fill if necessary. Place shells on spaghetti sauce in dish.

Pour remaining sauce evenly over shells, covering completely. Sprinkle with cheese.

Cover and bake about 1 1/2hours or until shells are tender.

Sprinkle with basil. 7servings 9 points Serve with a salad or any 0 pt.

# VeggiesLinguine and Shrimp

1.2 cup Italian dressing (Fat-free)
1 clove garlic, minced
1/4 cup chopped parsley
2 tsp grated lemon peel
1 tsp salt
dash cayenne pepper
12 ounces shrimp
2 med. yellow squash, julienned
1 med. zucchini, julienned
1 med. carrot julienned
3 green onions
1/2 lb linguine, cooked

In medium skillet, heat Italian dressing and spices. Add all other ingredients except Linguine and sauté. Toss Linguine with vegetables, shrimp, and sauce. Serve at once.

This dish is not only delicious, it's a feast for the eyes. The bright vegetables tossed with pink shrimp and pasta look wonderful in a big serving bowl set in the middle of the dinner table. Double or even triple the recipe, add simple salad and crust bread, and you can easily feed a crowd.

Four BIG servings, 5.5 points each

# Pasta e fagioli (pasta and beans)

1 (16 oz) can Italian-style crushed or whole Italian-style tomatoes (finely chopped)
1 (19 oz) can kidney or cannellini beans, rinsed and drained
1 cup frozen mixed vegetables
3 cups cooked pasta or 3/4 cup dry pasta
3 cups water

Place all ingredients in a medium-size saucepan

Simmer 10 minutes, if using cooked pasta, or until dry pasta is fully cooked. Add enough water during cooking to just cover the pasta.

4 servings, 3 points each

# Pizza

## *Homemade Pizza*

### Dough

1 pkg yeast
1 c. warm water
1 T. sugar
2 T. oil
1 t. salt
1 t. Italian seasoning
1 t. garlic powder
3 c. flour

### Topping

1/2 c. pizza sauce 1/4 c mushroom 1/4 c. onions
2 T. pimento
1/2 c. tiny shrimp
1/2 c. low fat cheddar
1/2 c. lpw fatf mozzarella

Dissolve yeast in warm water. Stir in sugar, oil, salt and 1 c. flour. Add Italian seasoning and garlic. Beat until smooth. Mix in enough flour to make dough easy to handle. Knead about 5 minutes. Place in sprayed bowl and let rise until double (30 min). Form dough into pizza pan and bake 10 min @ 350 deg.

Add topping. Bake until cheese is melted and crust is brown. If using fat free cheese, cover during second baking.

Variations limited only by imagination. 8 servings, 4 points each

# Fireworks Pizza

1 package (10 oz) thin Italian bread shell or ready to serve pizza crust (12 - 14 inches in diameter)
1 jar (12 oz) gardiniera vegetable mix (found in the pickle section of grocery store. Contains carrots, broccoli, cauliflower, etc.), drained
1 tablespoon chopped drained pepperoncini peppers ( I used red bell peppers)
3/4 cup crumbled feta cheese
2 teaspoons chopped fresh parsley

Heat oven to 400.

Place bread shell on ungreased cookie sheet. Mix vegetable mix and pepper, spread evenly over bread shell. Sprinkle with cheese and parsley.

Bake 10 to 12 minutes or until cheese is melted and bubbly.

8 servings, 4 points each

# Lite Muffin Pizzas

Lite muffins
Fat fee cheese (1 point per slice)
Parsley, garlic powder (optional).
Tiny bit of salt.
Black pepper, onions, tomatoes.

Pre-heat oven to 350

Cut up the onions, and tomatoes how you like them. Then in a medium bowl mix them with just a tiny bit of oil, parsley, black pepper and if you like garlic powder.

Cut muffins in half and put the stuff in bowl on top of muffins. Put on a cookie sheet and bake to your liking. My friends like it where the bottom is black. I like it when it is a bit golden. For the cheese there is two ways you can do this. I take out the muffins and put a half of the slice on each one and put back in oven for a few minutes until melted.

Take out the muffins and put the half of slice on each and let it melt.

1 whole muffin is 2 points. Half of the muffin is only one point.

# Poultry

## *Chicken Parmigiana*

1/3 cup all purpose flour
1/4 teaspoon garlic powder
1/4 teaspoon paprika
1/4 teaspoon pepper
6 (4 oz) skinless, boneless chicken breast halves
2 large egg whites, lightly beaten
2 cups corn-flakes, coarsely crushed Cooking spray
1 (26 oz) jar low-fat spaghetti sauce
3/4 cup (3 oz) shredded part-skim mozzarella cheese

Preheat oven to 350 degrees.

Combine first 4 ingredients in a shallow dish. Dredge each piece of chicken in flour mixture. Dip each piece of chicken in egg whites; dredge in corn flakes. Arrange chicken in a 13 x 9-inch baking dish coated with cooking spray. Bake at 350 for 25 minutes or until crisp.

Place spaghetti sauce in a medium saucepan, and cook over medium heat until thoroughly heated. Pour sauce over chicken and sprinkle with mozzarella cheese.

Bake an additional 5 minutes or until cheese melts.

Serving size is 1 chicken breast half and 1/2 cup sauce.

6 servings, 5 points each

# Cheesy Chicken Rolls

1 tablespoon chives
1 tablespoon lowfat yogurt -- plain
1 tablespoon parsley
1/4 cup lowfat yogurt -- plain
2 1/2 cups mushroom -- sliced
1 tablespoon pimientos -- cut into strips
1 pound skinless boneless chicken breast
1 tablespoon bread crumbs -- fine
1/2 cup lowfat mozzarella cheese -- shredded
1/8 teaspoon paprika

For filling, in a small bowl combine cheese, mushrooms, the 1/4 cup yogurt, chives, parsley, and pimento. Place 1 chicken breast half, boned side up, between 2 pieces of clear plastic wrap. Working from the center to the edges, pound lightly with a meat mallet to 1/8" thickness. Remove plastic wrap. Repeat with remaining chicken. Sprinkle lightly with salt and pepper. Spread some of the filling on each chicken breast half. Fold in the sides and roll up. Arrange rolls seam side down in a 10x6x2" baking dish.

Combine bread crumbs and paprika. Brush chicken with the 1 tablespoon yogurt; sprinkle with crumb mixture.

Bake in 350 degrees F. oven for 20-25 minutes or till chicken is tender and no longer pink.

4 servings, 4 points each

# Chicken Cordon Bleu

2 thin chicken cutlets (3 oz. each)
2 slices each turkey-ham and reduced-fat Swiss cheese (1 1/2 oz each)
1 Tablespoon plus 2 tsps. Dijon style mustard, divided
1 tsp. honey
1/3 c. plus 2 tsps. plain dried bread crumbs
2 tsps. vegetable oil
1/2 c. canned chicken broth
2 tsps. all purpose flour
1 Tablespoon sour cream

Preheat oven to 375 degrees. Top each chicken cutlet with 1 slice turkey ham and 1 slice cheese; starting from the narrow end, roll each cutlet jelly roll fashion. Secure with toothpicks. In small mixing bowl, combine 1 tablespoon mustard and the honey; spread half of the mixture evenly over each chicken roll.

On sheet of wax paper, arrange bread crumbs; turn chicken rolls in bread crumbs, coating all sides and using all of the bread crumbs. Arrange chicken rolls on nonstick baking sheet and drizzle each with 1 tsp. oil. Bake until chicken is cooked through, 20 to 25 minutes.

While chicken is baking, prepare sauce. In small saucepan, combine broth and flour; stirring to dissolve flour. Cook over medium-high heat, stirring frequently, until mixture thickens, 3 to 4 minutes. Reduce heat to low and stir in sour cream and remaining mustard; cook, stirring occasionally, 3 to 4 minutes longer (DO NOT BOIL).

To serve, remove toothpicks and cut each chicken roll crosswise into 4 equal slices. Onto each of 2 serving plates, pour half of the sauce ad top with 4 chicken roll slices.

Makes 2 servings, 7 points each

Approximate total time: 40 minutes (includes baking time).

# Chicken Stroganoff

1 pound frozen boneless skinless chicken breasts
1 can fat free cream of mushroom soup
16 oz. carton fat free sour cream
1 envelope dry onion soup mix

Put frozen chicken in bottom of crockpot.

Mix soup, sour cream, onion soup mix and pour over chicken.
Cook on low for 7 hours. (

Serve it over rice or noodles, but be sure to add those points)

6 servings, 4 points each

# Ginger Chicken

1 lb. boneless chicken breasts
1 Tbsp. veg. oil
2 cloves garlic
1 sweet green or red peppers cut in strips
1 cup thinly sliced mushrooms
2 Tbsp. each minced gingeroot and soy sauce
1 Tbsp. oyster sauce
1 tsp. granulated sugar
1/2 tsp. cornstarch
1/4 tsp. cayenne pepper
1/4 cup fresh coriander (cilantro)

Cut chicken into thin strips

In nonstick skillet heat oil over high heat and stir fry chicken and garlic for 2 min. Add sweet pepper and mushrooms and fry for 1 min.

Stir together ginger, soy sauce, oyster sauce, 1 Tbsp. water, sugar, cornstarch and cayenne pepper. Add to skillet and fry for 1 minute or until chicken is no longer pink inside and sauce is thickened. Sprinkle with cilantro.

Note: Cut down even further by sautéing the chicken and garlic in a little chicken broth instead of oil.

4 servings, 4 points each

# Chicken and Dumplings

4 skinless, boneless chicken breasts
5 fat free tortillas
2 c. low salt chicken broth
1 c. water
1/2 can evaporated skim milk
2 chicken bouillon cubes
1 c. sliced carrots
1 large onion
1 c. sliced celery

Boil chicken and vegetables in broth and water. Remove chicken and vegies. Cube chicken. Add bouillon cubes to broth and bring to a rolling boil. Tear tortillas into pieces into broth. Cook at rolling boil 5 minutes

Add evaporated skim milk, chicken, vegetables. Salt and pepper to taste. Cover and simmer until thick as you like (15 min)

Tortillas puff up to become dumplings. I think they are more like homemade noodles but great whatever you call them.

8, 1 cup servings, 3 points each

# Mexican Chicken Breasts

1 Pkg Taco seasoning (Taco Bell is best)
4 (4 oz) chicken breasts
1 cup salsa
1/4 cup non-fat sour cream

Put chicken in plastic bag; shake and coat well. Place in sprayed (nonstick cooking spray) casserole dish. Bake 30 minutes in a 375 oven. Top with salsa about 5 minutes before done, then top with sour cream.

Makes 4 servings, 4 points each

# Mexican Chicken Bake

28 tortilla chips
1 cup onion -- chopped
1 cup green peppers -- chopped
1 tbl chili powder
1 cup chicken breasts -- chopped
3/4 cup gravy (fat-free chicken Heinz) cup
1/4 cup cheddar cheese, low fat (Healthy Choice) -- shredded

Layer chips on the bottom of 8x8 pan. Cook onions, peppers & chilies for 3 minutes. Stir in tomatoes, chicken & gravy. Add to chips and bake at 350 for 30 min. Add cheese when done.

4 servings, 5 points each

# Ranch Chicken Stir Fry

1 Tbsp Vegetable oil
1/2 LB Chicken breast strips-boneless, skinless
1 package Ranch Salad Dressing Mix, Hidden Valley Oriinal
16 oz vegetable medley, thawed
2 Tbsp water

Heat vegetable oil in large skillet.

Add chicken breast strips.

Stir in one package Hidden Valley original ranch dressing mix to coat chicken.

 Add thawed vegetable medley and water.

Stir-fry about 2 minutes.

4 servings, 1.5 points each

# Chicken & Vegetable Stir Fry

1/3 cup Chicken Broth
2 Tbsp sherry
1 Tbsp Low Sodium Soy sauce
1/8 tsp black pepper
2 whole chicken breasts
1 Tbsp Peanut oil
6 oz frozen snow peas (drained)
1/4 LB mushrooms sliced
2 Tbsp chopped green pepper
2 Tbsp green onions
2 garlic cloves minced
1/4 tsp chopped ginger

In a shallow dish, combine chicken broth, sherry, soy sauce, cornstarch and pepper.

Split, skin and debone the chicken breasts. Cut into 1/2" pieces. Add to mix in pan. Toss well. Refrigerate for about an hour.

In a large skillet, over high heat, heat oil, add snow peas, mushrooms, onions, peppers, garlic and ginger and cook for about five minutes or until crisp.

Remove from skillet and set aside.

 Add chicken and marinade to skillet and cook for 10 minutes or until chicken is tender and sauce has thickened. If needed add 1/4 cup water to the skillet. Return vegetables to skillet.

Cook, stirring frequently about 2 minutes.

4 Servings, 2.5 points each

# Chicken Meat Loaf

1 1/2 lb ground chicken
1/2 cup finely chopped mushrooms
1/3 cup dry bread crumbs
1/4 cup milk
1 small onion, finely chopped
1 egg, lightly beaten
2 tbsp Dijon mustard
1 1/2 tsp Worcestershire Sauce
1/2 tsp salt
Black pepper to taste
1/4 cup Chili or Salsa Sauce

Preheat oven to 350F. Put all ingredients (except chili or salsa sauce) in a large bowl. Use your hands to mix just until blended. Pat into a 9x5x3-inch loaf pan, rounding the top slightly. Spread chili sauce over top of meat loaf.

Bake 1-1/4 to 1-1/2 hours, until meat juices run clear. Drain fat halfway through baking. It is very important that the meatloaf be cooked completely. Let meatloaf stand for 10 minutes before slicing.

3 points.

# Layered Chicken Dinner

1 c. uncooked regular rice
2 c. (16 oz can) cut green beans, drained
16 oz skinless, boneless chicken breast cut into 4 pieces
1 can Health Request Cream of Chicken
1/2 c. (2.5 oz jar) sliced mushrooms, drained
2 T. Bacon Bits
3/4 c. water
1 t. dried parsley flakes
1 t. dried onion flakes
1/4 t. black pepper

Preheat oven to 350 degrees. Spray 8 x 8 pan with butter flavored spray.

Layer rice, green beans, and chicken in prepared pan. In medium bowl, combine soup, mushrooms, bacon bits, water, parsley and onion flakes and pepper. Spoon evenly over.

Cover and bake 90 minutes. Uncover and continue baking 15 minutes

4 servings, 6 points each

# Stuffed Chicken Breast

1 skinless boneless chicken breast
1/4 pkg of frozen chopped spinach thawed
1/4 lb sliced mushrooms
3 Tbs grated low fat jack cheese
1 Tbs minced red onion

Pound chicken breast until even and thin between sheets of plastic wrap.

In a sauté pan sprayed with Pam, and a little olive oil, cook onions and mushrooms until soft, add spinach and sauté slightly, Add cheese and stir until melted.

Add filling to chicken breast and roll up or fold to enclose. (You will have left over filling.)

Brush chicken with a little olive oil and season with herbs of your choice and bake until browned.

NOTE: you can use as many chicken breasts as will hold the filling. These freeze wonderfully and can be baked frozen.

1 servings, 5 points

# Turkey Salsa Meat Loaf

1 TBSP olive oil
1 Cup finely chopped yellow onion (aobut 1 med-lg onion)
1/2 Cup finely chopped carrot (about 1 med-small carrot)
1/4 C finely chopped celery (about 1 small rib)
1 lb. extra lean ground turkey breast
1 cup old fashioned rolled oats (not quick cooking)
1/2 cup plus 3 TBSP nonfat tomato salsa (as hot as you like)
1 large egg
2 TSP minced fresh Italian (flat leaf)parsley
3/4 tsp. salt
1 tsp. freshly ground black pepper

Preheat oven to 375 degrees. Coat 8 1/2 x 4 1/2 x 2 3/4 inc. loaf pan with nonstick cooking spray and set aside.

Heat olive oil in med. size heavy skillet over moderately high heat for 1 min. Add onion, carrot and celery and stir fry until limp - about 5 minutes.

Transfer skillet mixture to large bowl. Add turkey, rolled oats, 1/2 c. salsa and all remaining ingredients. Mix well.

Pat mixture into prepared pan and bake uncovered 30 minutes. Spread remaining 3 TBSP salsa on top and bake until meatloaf is set and juices run clear- about 15 mins. longer.

Remove meatloaf from oven and let stand in upright pan 15 minutes; this firms up the loaf and allows the juices to settle.

Cut into six thick slices and serve.

Makes 6 servings at 4 pts apiece

# White Bean Chili

1Tbsp (or less) oil
1 lb chicken, cut in 1" pieces
1 medium onion, chopped
2 cloves garlic, minced
1 can (15 oz) diced tomatoes w/jalapenos
3 cans (15 oz each) small white beans, undrained
3 tbsp mesquite marinade sauce
1/4 cup chopped parsley or cilantro

Sauté garlic and onion in oil until soft. Add chicken and cook until no longer pink.

Reduce heat to low. Add the rest of the ingredients and simmer for 10 minutes or so.

Makes 6 servings, 4 points each

# White Chili

48 oz great northern beans (precooked)
3 chicken breasts
2 cup chicken broth
2 cups salsa, thick and chunky
1 cup mozzarella cheese, part skim, grated

Cook chicken until tender in water and reserve 2 cups broth or use canned. Cut up chicken, add other ingredients, and simmer for 1 hour. Serving size 1 cup.

2 points

# Salads and Dressings

## *Mexican Tuna Salad*

4 oz. drained canned tuna flaked
1/2 med. tomato, finely chopped
1/4 c. finely chopped red onion
1/4 c. finely chopped red pepper
2 Tablespoons plus 2 tsps. reduced calorie mayonnaise
1 Tablespoon each chopped cilantro or Italian parsley
1 Tablespoon lime juice

In small mixing bowl, combine all ingredients, mixing well.

Serve in a taco with shredded lettuce and diced tomato.

4 servings, 2 points each

## *Cranberry Salad*

20 oz can crushed pineapple
12 oz cranberries (chopped)
1 c. Lite cool whip
1 small pkg sugar free vanilla instant pudding

Drain pineapple, add juice to pudding mix. Stir in remaining ingredients. Chill.

Great holiday side dish.

# Creamy Potato Salad

3 cups peeled, cooked , cubed potatoes
2 T. chopped green onions
1 2 oz jar diced pimento, drained
1/4 c. fat free mayo
1/4 c. fat free yogurt
1 T. prepared mustard
1 1/2 t. each sugar and white vinegar
1/4 t. each salt and celery seed
1/8 t. each garlic powder and pepper

Combine potatoes, onions and pimento. Put sauce ingredients
in jar and shake to mix. Pour sauce over potatoes and mix well.
Refrigerate to blend flavors before serving.

6, 1/2 c. servings, 1 point each

# Sauces, Dips and Spreads

## *Alfredo Sauce*

1 cup skim milk
2 tablespoon flour
1 tablespoon Molly McButterä
1/2 teaspoon dried parsley
2 tablespoon grated Parmesan cheese salt & pepper

In a small jar with a tight lid, shake together the flour and skim milk. Pour into small saucepan. Add parsley, salt, and pepper. Simmer until thickened. Add Parmesan cheese. Serve over cooked pasta.

Makes 1 cup, enough for 2 cups of pasta, 3 points


## *Tomato-Herb Sauce*

4 tsp olive oil
12 plum (Roma) tomatoes
2 tb parsley, minced
2 tb basil, minced, or 1 tsp dried
1 tb oregano, minced, or 1 tsp dried
2 tsp thyme, minced, or 1/2 tsp dried
1 garlic clove, minced
1/4 tsp salt
Pepper to taste

Put half the tomatoes in a blender. Heat the oil in a nonstick saucepan, then add remaining ingredients. Cook, stirring frequently, until reduced to about 2 cups, about 15 minutes.

4 servings, 1 point each

# Snacks

## Chewy Oatmeal-Apricot Cookies

1 1/2 cups oatmeal -- uncooked
1 1/4 cups all-purpose flour
1 teaspoon baking soda
1/2 teaspoon baking powder
1 teaspoon cinnamon
1/2 teaspoon salt
1/4 teaspoon ground nutmeg
3/4 cup unsweetened applesauce
1/2 cup light brown sugar -- plus 2 tablespoons
2 large egg whites
2 tablespoons margarine -- melted
1 teaspoon vanilla extract
1 cup dried apricot halves – diced

Preheat the oven to 350 degrees.

Spray two large baking sheets with no-stick spray; set aside. Spread the rolled oats on an ungreased baking sheet and toast for 8-10 minutes until lightly browned. In a large mixing bowl, combine the toasted oats, flour, baking soda, cinnamon, baking powder, salt and nutmeg, stir well, set aside.

In another large mixing bowl, with an electric mixer at medium speed, beat the applesauce, brown sugar, egg whites, margarine and vanilla until well combined. With mixer at low speed, gradually beat in the dry ingredients until well combined. Stir in the apricots. Drop the dough by level tablespoons, 1 inch apart, onto the prepared baking sheets.

Place both sheets in the oven and bake for 10 to 12 minutes (switching the positions of the sheets halfway through baking), or until cookies are lightly browned. Transfer cookies to wire racks to cool.

42 servings, 1 point each

# *Peanut Butter Cookies*

3/4 cup creamy peanut butter
2 tablespoon margarine
1/3 cup + 2 teaspoon applesauce
1 1/4 cup flour
1/2 cup granulated sugar
1/2 cup brown sugar
egg
teaspoon baking soda
1/4 teaspoon baking powder dash of salt

Preheat oven to 350.

With mixer on medium combine peanut butter, margarine and applesauce. Add remaining ingredients and mix well. Roll dough into 1 inch balls and arrange 3 inches apart on non-stick cookie sheet. Make criss-cross pattern with fork. Bake 10-12 minutes. Cool on wire rack.

Makes 60 cookies, 1 point each

# Italian Popcorn

12 cups cooked popcorn
1 Tb cayenne pepper
1 Tb paprika
1 Tb chili pepper
2 tsp garlic powder

Mix seasonings together and sprinkle on popcorn as soon as it is popped. If using a hot-air popper, sprinkle it on as the popcorn shoots out.

6 servings, 1 point each

# Slow Cooker Party Snacks

1 1/2 Cups Keebler fat-free and reduced sodium coarsely broken pretzels (3 ounces)
2 Cups Wheat Chex
2 1/2 Cups Cheerios
2 1/2 Cups Rice Chex
1/2 Cup Dry Roasted Peanuts
1/4 Cup Grated Kraft Fat-Free Parmesan Cheese
1/4 Cup Kraft Fat-Free Italian Dressing

In a slow cooker container, combine pretzels, Wheat Chex,Cheerios, Rice Chex, peanuts and Parmesan Cheese.

Add Italian Dressing. Mix well to combine. Cover and cook on LOW for 4 hours. Uncover. Continue cooking on LOW 30 minutes, stirring occasionally.

12, 3/4 cup servings, 3 points each

# Soups and Stews

## *Soups*

### *Cauliflower Soup*

1 Head Cauliflower
4 teaspoon Garlic
2 tablespoon Olive Oil
1 large can Fat Free College Inn Chicken Broth
2 teaspoon Dried Italian Seasoning
4 tablespoon of good Parmesan Cheese
Salt and Pepper to taste

In a pot put oil and sauté garlic. Add cauliflower broken off stem and all other ingredients (except the cheese).

Cook 1 hour, then with the back of a wooden spoon break up all the cauliflower till it looks like small crumbles.

Shut off the stove, add cheese to pot and stir and serve.

2 points

# Garden Vegetable Soup

2/3 cup sliced carrot
1/2 cup diced onion
2 garlic cloves, minced
3 cup broth (beef, chicken or veggie)
1 1/2 cup diced green cabbage
1/2 cup green beans
1 tablespoon tomato paste
1/2 teaspoon dried basil
1/4 teaspoon dried oregano
1/4 teaspoon salt
1/2 cup diced zucchini

In a large saucepan sprayed with nonstick cooking spray, saute carrot, onion and garlic over low heat until softened, about 5 min. Add broth, cabbage, beans, tomato paste, basil, oregano and salt; bring to a boil. Lower heat and simmer, covered, about 15 min. or until beans are tender. Stir in zucchini and heat 3-4 min. Serve hot.

2 Points

# Italian Wedding Soup

1/2 pound ground beef, extra lean 1/2 pound ground veal
1/4 cup seasoned bread crumbs
1 egg
1 tablespoon parsley
salt and pepper to taste
4 cups chicken broth
2 cups spinach leaves, cut in tiny pieces
1/4 cup Romano cheese, grated

Combine the ground meat, breadcrumbs, egg, parsley, salt and pepper in a bowl. Mix well and form into tiny meatballs. Bake on a cookie sheet for 30 minutes at 350º. Meanwhile, bring broth to a boil and add spinach.

Cover and boil for 5 minutes. Add the meatballs to the hot broth, bring to a simmer. Stir in the cheese and serve immediately.

8 Servings, 4 points each

# Low-Fat Broccoli Soup

1 can (14.5 oz) low-sodium chicken broth
2 cups chopped fresh or frozen broccoli
1/2 cup chopped onion
2 tbsp cornstarch
1 can (12 oz) evaporated skim milk

In a saucepan, combine broccoli, onion and broth; simmer for 10 to 15 minutes or until vegetables are tender.

Puree half of the mixture in a blender; return to the saucepan. In a small bowl, whisk the cornstarch and 3 tbsp of milk until smooth. Gradually add remaining milk. Stir into the broccoli mixture. Bring to a boil; boil and stir for 2 minutes.

SERVING SIZE: 3/4 cup. 4 servings, 1 point each

# Cheese and Broccoli Soup

2 tsps. reduced calorie margarine (tub)
2 Tablespoons finely chopped onion
1 Tablespoon plus 1 1/2 tsps. all-purpose flour
1 c. water
1 c. skim or nonfat milk
1 c. broccoli florets
1 packet instant chicken broth and seasoning mix
1/2 tsp. chopped fresh parsley
Dash white pepper
3/4 oz. reduced fat Cheddar or Monterey Jack cheese, shredded

In 2 quart nonstick saucepan, melt margarine; add onion and sauté over medium high heat, until softened, 1 to 2 minutes. Sprinkle flour over onion and stir quickly to combine. Continuing to stir, add 1 cup water and the milk; add broccoli, broth mix, parsley and pepper.

Reduce heat to low and cook, stirring occasionally, until broccoli is tender, 10 to 15 minutes (do not boil). Let cool slightly.

In blender process half of the soup until smooth; return to saucepan. Stir in cheese and cook over low heat until cheese is melted, about 5 minutes.

Makes 2 servings, 3 points each.

# Cheesy Broccoli Soup

4 c water
12 oz shredded frozen hash brown potatoes
1 c chopped celery
1 c chopped onion

1 c chopped carrots
4 c chopped broccoli
2 pkts chicken broth
1 t salt
1.2 t pepper
3 T flour
2 c skim milk
6 oz Velveeta cheese, cubed

Combine all the ingredients except the flour, milk & cheese in a large pot and bring to a boil. Simmer for 15-20 minutes Blend flour & milk. Slowly add to vegetables. Finally, add the cheese. Stir until melted.

4 servings, 5 points each

# New England Clam Chowder

2 slices bacon, cut into 1/2 inch pieces
1 medium onion, chopped (1/2 cup)
2 cans (6 1/2 oz. each) minced clams, drained and liquid
reserved 2 medium, potatoes, diced (2 cups)
dash of pepper
2 cups skim milk

Cook bacon and onion in 2-quart saucepan over medium-high heat, stirring frequently, until bacon is crisp.

Add enough water, if necessary, to reserved clam liquid to measure 1 cup. Stir clams, clam liquid, potatoes and pepper into onion mixture. Heat to boiling; reduce heat to medium. Cover and cook about 15 minutes or until potatoes are tender. Stir in milk.

Heat stirring occasionally, just until hot (do not boil). 4 Servings, 4 points each

# Light Lentil Soup

1 lb. carrots, peeled and sliced
1 large onion, chopped
2 15-17oz. cans Italian style stewed tomatoes
1 lb. lentils, rinsed and drained
2 cloves garlic, minced
2 teaspoon of leaf thyme
1 1/2 teaspoon salt
1 teaspoon black pepper
2-3 bay leaves
10 cups water

Low boil everything in a big pot (like a 5-qt. Dutch oven) for 30-40 minutes.

4 servings, 2 points each

# Mexican Vegetable Beef Soup

8 ounces ground turkey
1 cup onion, chopped
2 cups tomatoes, chopped
1 3/4 cups beef broth, 15 oz. can
1 3/4 cups tomato sauce, 15 oz. can
1 1/2 cups celery, diced
1 1/2 cups carrot, sliced
1 1/2 cups green beans, cut up
2 teaspoons chili seasoning mix
3/4 cup corn whole kernel, canned
6 ounces red kidney beans, canned, rinsed and drained
1 teaspoon parsley, flaked

In a large saucepan sprayed with butter-flavored cooking spray, brown meat and onion.

Stir in undrained tomatoes, beef broth and tomato sauce. Bring mixture to a boil. Add celery, carrots, green beans, chili seasoning mix, corn, kidney beans and parsley flakes. Mix well to combine. Lower heat, cover and simmer for 30 minutes or until vegetables are tender.

3 points

# Mushroom Soup

1 lb fresh mushrooms/ sliced
1/4 c. chopped onions
1 small clove garlic, minced
1/2 t. salt
1/4 t. Worcestershire sauce
1/2 t. dry mustard
3 T. sherry or red wine
1 c. water
1 T. flour
1/2 c. chopped celery
1 t. parsley flakes
1 medium potato
1/2 c. carrots, shredded
2 c. beef broth (1 T granules + 2 c. water)

Melt 1 T butter in Dutch oven and add onion and garlic. Cook until tender. Blend in salt,

Worchestershire sauce, dry mustard and flour. Slowly add beef broth, wine and water. Bring to a boil, add celery, parsley, carrots, potatoes and mushrooms. Cover and simmer 30 minutes.

4-6, 1 cup servings, 1.25 points each

# Potato Soup

Serving Size : 6 Preparation Time :0:00 4 cups potatoes -- thinly sliced
1 medium onion -- diced
3 tablespoons butter
1 1/2 cups potato water
1 1/2 cups evaporated skim milk
1 teaspoon salt
4 teaspoons minced parsley -- optional chopped chives -- optional

Peel, wash and slice potatoes and add onions and enough water to just cover. Cook covered for 15 minutes.

Drain and reserve 1 1/2 cups of potato water. Mash potatoes, add butter, water milk and salt. Heat very good. If desired top each serving with a teaspoon of minced parsley or chopped chives

6 servings, 4 points each

# Taco Soup

1 lb. lean hamburger meat
1 cup onion, chopped
3 16 oz cans chili or pinto beans (not drained)
1 can of whole kernel corn (not drained)
1 can diced tomatoes (optional)
1 can peppers (optional)
1 8 oz. Can tomato sauce
1 package Taco seasoning
1 package Hidden Valley Ranch dressing mix (Do not mix the dressing. Use it dry.)
1 1/2 cups water

Fry the hamburger and onion, drain off the excess grease. Combine all other ingredients, and add water to desired.

Consistency, about 1 1/2 cups and simmer for 20 minutes. This recipe will freeze for three months.

Makes 12, 1 cup servings, 3 points each

# Stews

## Italian Seafood Stew

2 c. sliced carrots (1 inch pieces)
1 c. canned Italian tomatoes (with liquid), pureed
3 ozs. diced pared potato
1/2 c. diced leeks (some green and some white portion)
1/4 c. dry white table wine
2 tsp. all purpose flour
2 garlic cloves, minced
1/4 lb. each sea scallops and shelled, deveined large shrimp
2 bay leaves
1/4 tsp. fennel seed
1/8 tsp. crushed red pepper

In 3 quart microwaveable casserole dish combine 1/2 cups water, carrots, tomatoes, potato, leeks, wine, flour and garlic, stirring to dissolve flour. Cover and microwave on High (100%) for 10 minutes, until carrots are tender.

Add scallops, shrimp and bay leaves; cover and microwave on High for 3 minutes until shrimp is pink.

Add fennel seed and pepper and stir to combine. Remove and discard bay leaves. Makes 2 servings, 4 points each.

Approximate total time: 25 minutes

# Vegetable Dishes

## *Garlic 'N' Onion Mashed Potatoes*

9 oz. pared potatoes, cubed
1/4 c. diced onion
1 1/2 garlic cloves, chopped
1/4 c. evaporated skimmed milk
2 tsps. margarine
dash white pepper

In 2 quart saucepan, bring 1 1/2 quarts of water to a boil; add potatoes, onion and garlic and cook until potatoes are fork tender, 10 to 15 minutes.

While potatoes are cooking, prepare milk mixture. In small nonstick saucepan, combine milk, margarine and pepper and cook over low heat until margarine is melted. Keep warm over low heat.

Pour potato-onion mixture through colander, discarding cooking liquid. Transfer potato-onion mixture to large mixing bowl. Using mixer on low speed, mash potato-onion mixture. Gradually increase speed to high; add milk mixture and continue beating until potatoes are light and fluffy.

Makes 2 servings, 3 points each.

# Spinach Pie

2 teaspoon oil
2 10 ounce packages fresh (or frozen) spinach, cleaned and coarsely chopped (or thawed and drained)
12 scallions, sliced
3/4 cups crumbled feta cheese
2/3 cup low-fat cottage cheese
1/2 cup minced dill
2 eggs, lightly beaten
14 teaspoon freshly ground black pepper
6 sheets phyllo dough, thawed if frozen

Preheat the oven to 350. Spray an 8" square baking pan with nonstick cooking spray. In a medium nonstick skillet, heat the oil. Add the scallions; cook, stirring, 1 minute. Add the spinach; cook, stirring as needed, until just wilted. 3-5 minutes. Transfer to a medium bowl; stir in the cheeses, dill, eggs and pepper.

Spray 1 phyllo sheet with nonstick cooking spray; top with another sheet and spray it.

Line the baking pan with these 2 sheets, letting the edges hang over the sides. Spread the spinach mixture over the phyllo.

Cover the filling with the remaining 4 sheets, spraying each sheet and tucking them into the pan, fold in the outside sheets.

Bake until golden, 30-35 minutes.

Makes 4 servings - 5 points each

# Onion Bloom

Amount Measure Ingredient -- Preparation Method
1 large onion
1/4 ounce corn flakes -- crumbled
1 pinch red pepper
1 pinch seasoned salt
1 egg white
1/2 cup nonfat sour cream
2 teaspoons Miracle Whip® light
1 teaspoon horseradish sauce
1/2 clove garlic -- finely minced
Cooking spray

Preheat oven to 350 degrees F. Spray 2-cup round baking dish with cooking spray.

Trim root end of onion so it stands upright. Slice off 1/2" from top and remove peel.

With sharp knife, cut triangular slices to center of onion, slicing from top down and stopping 1/2" from bottom. Work your way around to make several "petals." Spray with cooking spray and place in microwaveable safe bowl. Cover and microwave on high for 3-4 minutes or until onion is slightly tender and petals have begun to separate.

In small bowl combine corn flake crumbs, seasoned salt, and pepper; set aside. In medium bowl, whip egg white until foamy. Dip onion in egg white, coating petals thoroughly. Place in prepared baking dish and sprinkle evenly with corn flake mixture.

Bake until lightly browned and crisp about 10-12 minutes. Meanwhile, combine sour cream, Miracle Whip, horseradish sauce and garlic. Cover and chill. This may be prepared up to 2 days ahead.

2 servings, 3 points each

# Spaghetti Squash Alfredo

1 medium spaghetti squash
1 cup sour cream, reduced fat
1/2 cup mozzarella cheese, part skim milk
1/4 cup grated Parmesan cheese
1/4 tsp. garlic powder
1/4 tsp. salt
1/4 tsp. black pepper

Split squash in half. Scoop out all of the seeds and lay it face down on a cookie sheet with a little water in the pan.

Bake at 350 degrees for about 45 minutes to an hour until you can squeeze it on the top and it starts to become tender. When done scrape out the inside of the squash with a fork, shredding it into noodle-like strands.

In a medium-sized saucepan, combine the remaining ingredients over medium -low heat and whisk until smooth and creamy, stirring frequently to prevent burning. Add the cood squash to the sauce and stir until thoroughly mixed and heated through. Serve immediately.

NOTE: If you want to save some time, cut the raw squash in half lengthwise and place in a microwave-safe covered casserole dish with 2 Tbsp. water; microwave for 10 to 12 minutes, or until tender. But be careful with cutting raw spaghetti squash. The outer skin is very hard.

6 servings, 3 points each

# Freshly Broiled Eggplant

1/2 c. finely chopped plum tomato
3 tb balsamic vinegar
2 tb chopped fresh basil
1 sm garlic clove, minced
1 sm eggplant (about 12 oz), cut into 1/2" slices
1/4 tsp salt
1/4 tsp pepper

Preheat broiler. Spray broiler rack with nonstick cooking spray.

In small bowl, whisk together tomato, vinegar, basil, & garlic. Arrange eggplant slices on prepared rack; brush slices with some of the tomato mixture.

Broil 5-6" from heat 8 minutes, until lightly browned. Turn slices, brush with more of the tomato mixture. Broil 3-5 minutes, until lightly browned. Transfer slices to serving bowl; keep warm.

Add salt & pepper to remaining tomato mixture; stir to combine. To serve, pour remaining tomato mixture over eggplant slices.

4 servings, 0 points

# Two Potato Scallop

3 cups each sliced peeled sweet and white potato
2 large cloves garlic, minced
1/3 cup freshly grated Parmesan cheese
2 Tbsp. all purpose flour
1/4 tsp. each of salt, pepper and dried thyme
1 1/2 cups chicken or vegetable stock

In large bowl, mix together sweet and white potatoes, garlic, cheese, flour, salt, pepper and thyme. Transfer to 8 inch square pan sprayed with nonstick cooking spray.

Pour in stock. Cover with foil and bake in 375 degree oven for 50 minutes. Uncover and bake for 30 to 40 minutes longer or until golden brown and potatoes are tender.

6 servings, 5 points each (Serve with 1 slice of ham - 3 points)

# Helpful Hints

## *Determining Portions in a Recipe*

To determine portion size of your recipe if it doesn't indicate it, put your final product in an oblong or square baking dish, then when you take it out of the oven you can cut it into equal size servings. If the recipe says it makes 8 servings, cut it into 8 pieces before serving, if it says 6 servings cut it into 6 servings and so on. This is a very quick and easy way to manage portion sizes.

Also, if a recipe is for a soup then most all recipe portions is for 1 cup.

# Alphabetical List of Number of Calories Found in Specific Foods

SORTED BY FOOD NAME

| Description of food | | Fat (Grams) | Food Energy (calories) | Carbohydrate (Grams) | Protein (Grams) | Cholesterol (Milligrams) | Weight (Grams) | Saturated Fat (Grams) |
|---|---|---|---|---|---|---|---|---|
| 1000 ISLAND, SALAD DRSNG,LOCAL | 1 TBSP | 2 | 25 | 2 | 0 | 2 | 15 | 0.2 |
| 1000 ISLAND, SALAD DRSNG,REGLR | 1 TBSP | 6 | 60 | 2 | 0 | 4 | 16 | 1 |
| 100% NATURAL CEREAL | 1 OZ | 6 | 135 | 18 | 3 | 0 | 28.35 | 4.1 |
| 40% BRAN FLAKES, KELLOGG'S | 1 OZ | 1 | 90 | 22 | 4 | 0 | 28.35 | 0.1 |
| 40% BRAN FLAKES, POST | 1 OZ | 0 | 90 | 22 | 3 | 0 | 28.35 | 0.1 |
| ALFALFA SEEDS, SPROUTED, RAW | 1 CUP | 0 | 10 | 1 | 1 | 0 | 33 | 0 |
| ALL-BRAN CEREAL | 1 OZ | 1 | 70 | 21 | 4 | 0 | 28.35 | 0.1 |
| ALMONDS, SLIVERED | 1 CUP | 70 | 795 | 28 | 27 | 0 | 135 | 6.7 |
| ALMONDS, WHOLE | 1 OZ | 15 | 165 | 6 | 6 | 0 | 28.35 | 1.4 |
| ANGELFOOD CAKE, FROM MIX | 1 CAKE | 2 | 1510 | 342 | 38 | 0 | 635 | 0.4 |
| ANGELFOOD CAKE, FROM MIX | 1 PIECE | 0 | 125 | 29 | 3 | 0 | 53 | 0 |
| APPLE JUICE, CANNED | 1 CUP | 0 | 115 | 29 | 0 | 0 | 248 | 0 |
| APPLE PIE | 1 PIE | 105 | 2420 | 360 | 21 | 0 | 945 | 27.4 |

Description of food

| Description of food | | Fat (Grams) | Food Energy (calories) | Carbohydrate (Grams) | Protein (Grams) | Cholesterol (Milligrams) | Weight (Grams) | Saturated Fat (Grams) |
|---|---|---|---|---|---|---|---|---|
| APPLE PIE | 1 PIECE | 18 | 405 | 60 | 3 | 0 | 158 | 4.6 |
| APPLESAUCE, CANNED, SWEETENED | 1 CUP | 0 | 195 | 51 | 0 | 0 | 255 | 0.1 |
| APPLESAUCE, CANNED,UNSWEETENED | 1 CUP | 0 | 105 | 28 | 0 | 0 | 244 | 0 |
| APPLES, DRIED, SULFURED | 10 RINGS | 0 | 155 | 42 | 1 | 0 | 64 | 0 |
| APPLES, RAW, PEELED, SLICED | 1 CUP | 0 | 65 | 16 | 0 | 0 | 110 | 0.1 |
| APPLES, RAW, UNPEELED,2 PER LB | 1 APPLE | 1 | 125 | 32 | 0 | 0 | 212 | 0.1 |
| APPLES, RAW, UNPEELED,3 PER LB | 1 APPLE | 0 | 80 | 21 | 0 | 0 | 138 | 0.1 |
| APRICOT NECTAR, NO ADDED VIT C | 1 CUP | 0 | 140 | 36 | 1 | 0 | 251 | 0 |
| APRICOTS, CANNED, JUICE PACK | 1 CUP | 0 | 120 | 31 | 2 | 0 | 248 | 0 |
| APRICOTS, CANNED, JUICE PACK | 3 HALVES | 0 | 40 | 10 | 1 | 0 | 84 | 0 |
| APRICOTS, DRIED, COOKED,UNSWTN | 1 CUP | 0 | 210 | 55 | 3 | 0 | 250 | 0 |
| APRICOTS, DRIED, UNCOOKED | 1 CUP | 1 | 310 | 80 | 5 | 0 | 130 | 0 |
| APRICOTS, RAW | 3 APRCOT | 0 | 50 | 12 | 1 | 0 | 106 | 0 |
| APRICOT, CANNED, HEAVY SYRUP | 1 CUP | 0 | 215 | 55 | 1 | 0 | 258 | 0 |
| APRICOT, CANNED, HEAVY SYRUP | 3 HALVES | 0 | 70 | 18 | 0 | 0 | 85 | 0 |
| ARTICHOKES, GLOBE, COOKED, DRN | 1 ARTCHK | 0 | 55 | 12 | 3 | 0 | 120 | 0 |
| ASPARAGUS, CKD FRM FRZ,DRN,CUT | 1 CUP | 1 | 50 | 9 | 5 | 0 | 180 | 0.2 |
| ASPARAGUS, CKD FRM FRZ,DR,SPER | 4 SPEARS | 0 | 15 | 3 | 2 | 0 | 60 | 0.1 |
| ASPARAGUS, CKD FRM RAW, DR,CUT | 1 CUP | 1 | 45 | 8 | 5 | 0 | 180 | 0.1 |
| ASPARAGUS, CKD FRM RAW,DR,SPER | 4 SPEARS | 0 | 15 | 3 | 2 | 0 | 60 | 0 |
| ASPARAGUS,CANNED,SPEARS,NOSALT | 4 SPEARS | 0 | 10 | 2 | 1 | 0 | 80 | 0 |
| ASPARAGUS,CANNED,SPEARS,W/SALT | 4 SPEARS | 0 | 10 | 2 | 1 | 0 | 80 | 0 |
| AVOCADOS, CALIFORNIA | 1 AVOCDO | 30 | 305 | 12 | 4 | 0 | 173 | 4.5 |
| AVOCADOS, FLORIDA | 1 AVOCDO | 27 | 340 | 27 | 5 | 0 | 304 | 5.3 |
| BAGELS, EGG | 1 BAGEL | 2 | 200 | 38 | 7 | 44 | 68 | 0.3 |

| Description of food | Fat (Grams) | Food Energy (calories) | Carbohydrate (Grams) | Protein (Grams) | Cholesterol (Milligrams) | Weight (Grams) | Saturated Fat (Grams) |
|---|---|---|---|---|---|---|---|
| BAGELS, PLAIN 1 BAGEL | 2 | 200 | 38 | 7 | 0 | 68 | 0.3 |
| BAKING POWDER, LOW SODIUM 1 TSP | 0 | 5 | 1 | 0 | 0 | 4.3 | 0 |
| BAKING POWDER, STRGHT PHOSPHAT1 TSP | 0 | 5 | 1 | 0 | 0 | 3.8 | 0 |
| BAKING POWDER,SAS, CA PO4 1 TSP | 0 | 5 | 1 | 0 | 0 | 3 | 0 |
| BAKING POWDER,SAS,CAPO4+CASO4 1 TSP | 0 | 5 | 1 | 0 | 0 | 2.9 | 0 |
| BAKING PWDR BISCUITS,FROM MIX 1 BISCUT | 3 | 95 | 14 | 2 | 0 | 28 | 0.8 |
| BAKING PWDR BISCUITS,HOMERECPE1 BISCUT | 5 | 100 | 13 | 2 | 0 | 28 | 1.2 |
| BAKING PWDR BISCUITS,REFRGDOGH1 BISCUT | 2 | 65 | 10 | 1 | 1 | 20 | 0.6 |
| BAMBOO SHOOTS, CANNED, DRAINED1 CUP | 1 | 25 | 4 | 2 | 0 | 131 | 0.1 |
| BANANAS 1 BANANA | 1 | 105 | 27 | 1 | 0 | 114 | 0.2 |
| BANANAS, SLICED 1 CUP | 1 | 140 | 35 | 2 | 0 | 150 | 0.3 |
| BARBECUE SAUCE 1 TBSP | 0 | 10 | 2 | 0 | 0 | 16 | 0 |
| BARLEY, PEARLED,LIGHT, UNCOOKD1 CUP | 2 | 700 | 158 | 16 | 0 | 200 | 0.3 |
| BEAN SPROUTS, MUNG, COOKD,DRAN1 CUP | 0 | 25 | 5 | 3 | 0 | 124 | 0 |
| BEAN SPROUTS, MUNG, RAW 1 CUP | 0 | 30 | 6 | 3 | 0 | 104 | 0 |
| BEAN WITH BACON SOUP, CANNED 1 CUP | 6 | 170 | 23 | 8 | 3 | 253 | 1.5 |
| BEANS,DRY,CANNED,W/FRANKFURTER1 CUP | 18 | 365 | 32 | 19 | 30 | 255 | 7.4 |
| BEANS,DRY,CANNED,W/PORK+SWTSCE1 CUP | 12 | 385 | 54 | 16 | 10 | 255 | 4.3 |
| BEANS,DRY,CANNED,W/PORK+TOMSCE1 CUP | 7 | 310 | 48 | 16 | 10 | 255 | 2.4 |
| BEEF AND VEGETABLE STEW,HM RCP1 CUP | 11 | 220 | 15 | 16 | 71 | 245 | 4.4 |
| BEEF BROTH, BOULLN, CONSM,CNND1 CUP | 1 | 15 | 0 | 3 | 0 | 240 | 0.3 |
| BEEF GRAVY, CANNED 1 CUP | 5 | 125 | 11 | 9 | 7 | 233 | 2.7 |
| BEEF HEART, BRAISED 3 OZ | 5 | 150 | 0 | 24 | 164 | 85 | 1.2 |
| BEEF LIVER, FRIED 3 OZ | 7 | 185 | 7 | 23 | 410 | 85 | 2.5 |
| BEEF NOODLE SOUP, CANNED 1 CUP | 3 | 85 | 9 | 5 | 5 | 244 | 1.1 |

| Description of food | Fat (Grams) | Food Energy (calories) | Carbohydrate (Grams) | Protein (Grams) | Cholesterol (Milligrams) | Weight (Grams) | Saturated Fat (Grams) |
|---|---|---|---|---|---|---|---|
| BEEF POTPIE, HOME RECIPE 1 PIECE | 30 | 515 | 39 | 21 | 42 | 210 | 7.9 |
| BEEF ROAST, EYE O RND, LEAN 2.6 OZ | 5 | 135 | 0 | 22 | 52 | 75 | 1.9 |
| BEEF ROAST, EYE O RND,LEAN+FAT3 OZ | 12 | 205 | 0 | 23 | 62 | 85 | 4.9 |
| BEEF ROAST, RIB, LEAN ONLY 2.2 OZ | 9 | 150 | 0 | 17 | 49 | 61 | 3.6 |
| BEEF ROAST, RIB, LEAN + FAT 3 OZ | 26 | 315 | 0 | 19 | 72 | 85 | 10.8 |
| BEEF STEAK,SIRLOIN,BROIL,LEAN 2.5 OZ | 6 | 150 | 0 | 22 | 64 | 72 | 2.6 |
| BEEF STEAK,SIRLOIN,BROIL,LN+FT3 OZ | 15 | 240 | 0 | 23 | 77 | 85 | 6.4 |
| BEEF, CANNED, CORNED 3 OZ | 10 | 185 | 0 | 22 | 80 | 85 | 4.2 |
| BEEF, CKD,BTTM ROUND,LEAN ONLY2.8 OZ | 8 | 175 | 0 | 25 | 75 | 78 | 2.7 |
| BEEF, CKD,BTTM ROUND,LEAN+ FAT3 OZ | 13 | 220 | 0 | 25 | 81 | 85 | 4.8 |
| BEEF, CKD,CHUCK BLADE,LEANONLY2.2 OZ | 9 | 170 | 0 | 19 | 66 | 62 | 3.9 |
| BEEF, CKD,CHUCK BLADE,LEAN+FAT3 OZ | 26 | 325 | 0 | 22 | 87 | 85 | 10.8 |
| BEEF, DRIED, CHIPPED 2.5 OZ | 4 | 145 | 0 | 24 | 46 | 72 | 1.8 |
| BEER, LIGHT 12 FL OZ | 0 | 95 | 5 | 1 | 0 | 355 | 0 |
| BEER, REGULAR 12 FL OZ | 0 | 150 | 13 | 1 | 0 | 360 | 0 |
| BEET GREENS, COOKED, DRAINED 1 CUP | 0 | 40 | 8 | 4 | 0 | 144 | 0 |
| BEETS, CANNED, DRAINED,NO SALT1 CUP | 0 | 55 | 12 | 2 | 0 | 170 | 0 |
| BEETS, CANNED, DRAINED,W/ SALT1 CUP | 0 | 55 | 12 | 2 | 0 | 170 | 0 |
| BEETS, COOKED, DRAINED, DICED 1 CUP | 0 | 55 | 11 | 2 | 0 | 170 | 0 |
| BEETS, COOKED, DRAINED, WHOLE 2 BEETS | 0 | 30 | 7 | 1 | 0 | 100 | 0 |
| BLACK-EYED PEAS, DRY, COOKED 1 CUP | 1 | 190 | 35 | 13 | 0 | 250 | 0.2 |
| BLACK BEANS, DRY, COOKED,DRAND1 CUP | 1 | 225 | 41 | 15 | 0 | 171 | 0.1 |
| BLACKBERRIES, RAW 1 CUP | 1 | 75 | 18 | 1 | 0 | 144 | 0.2 |
| BLACKEYE PEAS, IMMATR,RAW,CKED1 CUP | 1 | 180 | 30 | 13 | 0 | 165 | 0.3 |
| BLACKEYE PEAS, IMMTR,FRZN,CKED 1 CUP | 1 | 225 | 40 | 14 | 0 | 170 | 0.3 |

| Description of food | Fat (Grams) | Food Energy (calories) | Carbohydrate (Grams) | Protein (Grams) | Cholesterol (Milligrams) | Weight (Grams) | Saturated Fat (Grams) |
|---|---|---|---|---|---|---|---|
| BLUE CHEESE 1 OZ | 8 | 100 | 1 | 6 | 21 | 28.35 | 5.3 |
| BLUE CHEESE SALAD DRESSING 1 TBSP | 8 | 75 | 1 | 1 | 3 | 15 | 1.5 |
| BLUEBERRIES, FROZEN, SWEETENED1 CUP | 0 | 185 | 50 | 1 | 0 | 230 | 0 |
| BLUEBERRIES, FROZEN, SWEETENED10 OZ | 0 | 230 | 62 | 1 | 0 | 284 | 0 |
| BLUEBERRIES, RAW 1 CUP | 1 | 80 | 20 | 1 | 0 | 145 | 0 |
| BLUEBERRY MUFFINS, HOME RECIPE1 MUFFIN | 5 | 135 | 20 | 3 | 19 | 45 | 1.5 |
| BLUEBERRY MUFFINS,FROM COM MIX1 MUFFIN | 5 | 140 | 22 | 3 | 45 | 45 | 1.4 |
| BLUEBERRY PIE 1 PIE | 102 | 2285 | 330 | 23 | 0 | 945 | 25.5 |
| BLUEBERRY PIE 1 PIECE | 17 | 380 | 55 | 4 | 0 | 158 | 4.3 |
| BOLOGNA 2 SLICES | 16 | 180 | 2 | 7 | 31 | 57 | 6.1 |
| BOSTON BROWN BREAD,W/WHTECRNM 1 SLICE | 1 | 95 | 21 | 2 | 3 | 45 | 0.3 |
| BOSTON BROWN BREAD,W/YLIWCRNML1 SLICE | 1 | 95 | 21 | 2 | 3 | 45 | 0.3 |
| BOUILLON, DEHYDRTD, UNPREPARED1 PKT | 1 | 15 | 1 | 1 | 1 | 6 | 0.3 |
| BRAN MUFFINS, FROM COMMERL MIX1 MUFFIN | 4 | 140 | 24 | 3 | 28 | 45 | 1.3 |
| BRAN MUFFINS, HOME RECIPE 1 MUFFIN | 6 | 125 | 19 | 3 | 24 | 45 | 1.4 |
| BRAUNSCHWEIGER 2 SLICES | 18 | 205 | 2 | 8 | 89 | 57 | 6.2 |
| BRAZIL NUTS 1 OZ | 19 | 185 | 4 | 4 | 0 | 28.35 | 4.6 |
| BREAD STUFFING,FROM MX,DRYTYPE1 CUP | 31 | 500 | 50 | 9 | 0 | 140 | 6.1 |
| BREAD STUFFING,FROM MX,MOIST 1 CUP | 26 | 420 | 40 | 9 | 67 | 203 | 5.3 |
| BREADCRUMBS, DRY, GRATED 1 CUP | 5 | 390 | 73 | 13 | 5 | 100 | 1.5 |
| BROCCOLI, FRZN, COOKED, DRANED1 CUP | 0 | 50 | 10 | 6 | 0 | 185 | 0 |
| BROCCOLI, FRZN, COOKED, DRANED1 PIECE | 0 | 10 | 2 | 1 | 0 | 30 | 0 |
| BROCCOLI, RAW 1 SPEAR | 1 | 40 | 8 | 4 | 0 | 151 | 0.1 |
| BROCCOLI, RAW, COOKED, DRAINED1 CUP | 0 | 45 | 9 | 5 | 0 | 155 | 0.1 |
| BROCCOLI, RAW, COOKED, DRAINED1 SPEAR | 1 | 50 | 10 | 5 | 0 | 180 | 0.1 |

101

**Description of food**

| Description of food | Fat (Grams) | Food Energy (calories) | Carbohydrate (Grams) | Protein (Grams) | Cholesterol (Milligrams) | Weight (Grams) | Saturated Fat (Grams) |
|---|---|---|---|---|---|---|---|
| BROWN AND SERVE SAUSAGE,BRWND 1 LINK | 5 | 50 | 0 | 2 | 9 | 13 | 1.7 |
| BROWN GRAVY FROM DRY MIX 1 CUP | 2 | 80 | 14 | 3 | 2 | 261 | 0.9 |
| BROWNIES W/ NUTS,FRM HOME RECP1 BROWNE | 6 | 95 | 11 | 1 | 18 | 20 | 1.4 |
| BROWNIES W/ NUTS,FRSTNG,CMMRCL1 BROWNE | 4 | 100 | 16 | 1 | 14 | 25 | 1.6 |
| BRUSSELS SPROUTS, FRZN, COOKED1 CUP | 1 | 65 | 13 | 6 | 0 | 155 | 0.1 |
| BRUSSELS SPROUTS, RAW, COOKED 1 CUP | 1 | 60 | 13 | 4 | 0 | 155 | 0.2 |
| BUCKWHEAT FLOUR, LIGHT, SIFTED1 CUP | 1 | 340 | 78 | 6 | 0 | 98 | 0.2 |
| BULGUR, UNCOOKED 1 CUP | 3 | 600 | 129 | 19 | 0 | 170 | 1.2 |
| BUTTERMILK, DRIED 1 CUP | 7 | 465 | 59 | 41 | 83 | 120 | 4.3 |
| BUTTERMILK, FLUID 1 CUP | 2 | 100 | 12 | 8 | 9 | 245 | 1.3 |
| BUTTER, SALTED 1 PAT | 4 | 35 | 0 | 0 | 11 | 5 | 2.5 |
| BUTTER, SALTED 1 TBSP | 11 | 100 | 0 | 0 | 31 | 14 | 7.1 |
| BUTTER, SALTED 1/2 CUP | 92 | 810 | 0 | 1 | 247 | 113 | 57.1 |
| BUTTER, UNSALTED 1 PAT | 4 | 35 | 0 | 0 | 11 | 5 | 2.5 |
| BUTTER, UNSALTED 1 TBSP | 11 | 100 | 0 | 0 | 31 | 14 | 7.1 |
| BUTTER, UNSALTED 1/2 CUP | 92 | 810 | 0 | 1 | 247 | 113 | 57.1 |
| CABBAGE, CHINESE, PAK-CHOI,CKD1 CUP | 0 | 20 | 3 | 3 | 0 | 170 | 0 |
| CABBAGE, CHINESE,PE-TSAI, RAW 1 CUP | 0 | 10 | 2 | 1 | 0 | 76 | 0 |
| CABBAGE, COMMON, COOKED, DRNED1 CUP | 0 | 30 | 7 | 1 | 0 | 150 | 0 |
| CABBAGE, COMMON, RAW 1 CUP | 0 | 15 | 4 | 1 | 0 | 70 | 0 |
| CABBAGE, RED, RAW 1 CUP | 0 | 20 | 4 | 1 | 0 | 70 | 0 |
| CABBAGE, SAVOY, RAW 1 CUP | 0 | 20 | 4 | 1 | 0 | 70 | 0 |
| CAKE OR PASTRY FLOUR, SIFTED 1 CUP | 1 | 350 | 76 | 7 | 0 | 96 | 0.1 |
| CAMEMBERT CHEESE 1 WEDGE | 9 | 115 | 0 | 8 | 27 | 38 | 5.8 |
| CANTALOUP, RAW 1/2 MELN | 1 | 95 | 22 | 2 | 0 | 267 | 0.1 |

| Description of food | | Fat (Grams) | Food Energy (calories) | Carbohydrate (Grams) | Protein (Grams) | Cholesterol (Milligrams) | Weight (Grams) | Saturated Fat (Grams) |
|---|---|---|---|---|---|---|---|---|
| CAP'N CRUNCH CEREAL | 1 OZ | 3 | 120 | 23 | 1 | 0 | 28.35 | 1.7 |
| CARAMELS, PLAIN OR CHOCOLATE | 1 OZ | 3 | 115 | 22 | 1 | 1 | 28.35 | 2.2 |
| CAROB FLOUR | 1 CUP | 0 | 255 | 126 | 6 | 0 | 140 | 0 |
| CARROT CAKE,CREMCHESE FRST,REC1 | CAKE | 328 | 6175 | 775 | 63 | 1183 | 1536 | 66 |
| CARROT CAKE,CREMCHESE FRST,REC1 | PIECE | 21 | 385 | 48 | 4 | 74 | 96 | 4.1 |
| CARROTS, CANNED, DRN, W/ SALT | 1 CUP | 0 | 35 | 8 | 1 | 0 | 146 | 0.1 |
| CARROTS, CANNED,DRND, W/O SALT1 | CUP | 0 | 35 | 8 | 1 | 0 | 146 | 0.1 |
| CARROTS, COOKED FROM FROZEN | 1 CUP | 0 | 55 | 12 | 2 | 0 | 146 | 0 |
| CARROTS, COOKED FROM RAW | 1 CUP | 0 | 70 | 16 | 2 | 0 | 156 | 0.1 |
| CARROTS, RAW, GRATED | 1 CUP | 0 | 45 | 11 | 1 | 0 | 110 | 0 |
| CARROTS, RAW, WHOLE | 1 CARROT | 0 | 30 | 7 | 1 | 0 | 72 | 0 |
| CASHEW NUTS, DRY ROASTD,SALTED1 | OZ | 13 | 165 | 9 | 4 | 0 | 28.35 | 2.6 |
| CASHEW NUTS, DRY ROASTD,UNSALT1 | CUP | 63 | 785 | 45 | 21 | 0 | 137 | 12.5 |
| CASHEW NUTS, DRY ROASTD,UNSALT1 | OZ | 13 | 165 | 9 | 4 | 0 | 28.35 | 2.6 |
| CASHEW NUTS, DRY ROASTED,SALTD1 | CUP | 63 | 785 | 45 | 21 | 0 | 137 | 12.5 |
| CASHEW NUTS, OIL ROASTD,SALTED1 | CUP | 63 | 750 | 37 | 21 | 0 | 130 | 12.4 |
| CASHEW NUTS, OIL ROASTD,SALTED1 | OZ | 14 | 165 | 8 | 5 | 0 | 28.35 | 2.7 |
| CASHEW NUTS, OIL ROASTD,UNSALT1 | CUP | 63 | 750 | 37 | 21 | 0 | 130 | 12.4 |
| CASHEW NUTS, OIL ROASTD,UNSALT1 | OZ | 14 | 165 | 8 | 5 | 0 | 28.35 | 2.7 |
| CATSUP | 1 CUP | 1 | 290 | 69 | 5 | 0 | 273 | 0.2 |
| CATSUP | 1 TBSP | 0 | 15 | 4 | 0 | 0 | 15 | 0 |
| CAULIFLOWER, COOKED FROM FROZN1 | CUP | 0 | 35 | 7 | 3 | 0 | 180 | 0.1 |
| CAULIFLOWER, COOKED FROM RAW | 1 CUP | 0 | 30 | 6 | 2 | 0 | 125 | 0 |
| CAULIFLOWER, RAW | 1 CUP | 0 | 25 | 5 | 2 | 0 | 100 | 0 |
| CELERY SEED | 1 TSP | 1 | 10 | 1 | 0 | 0 | 2 | 0 |

| Description of food | Fat (Grams) | Food Energy (calories) | Carbohydrate (Grams) | Protein (Grams) | Cholesterol (Milligrams) | Weight (Grams) | Saturated Fat (Grams) |
|---|---|---|---|---|---|---|---|
| CELERY, PASCAL TYPE, RAW,PIECE1 CUP | 0 | 20 | 4 | 1 | 0 | 120 | 0 |
| CELERY, PASCAL TYPE, RAW,STALK1 STALK | 0 | 5 | 1 | 0 | 0 | 40 | 0 |
| CHEDDAR CHEESE 1 CU IN | 6 | 70 | 0 | 4 | 18 | 17 | 3.6 |
| CHEDDAR CHEESE 1 OZ | 9 | 115 | 0 | 7 | 30 | 28.35 | 6 |
| CHEDDDAR CHEESE, SHREDDED 1 CUP | 37 | 455 | 1 | 28 | 119 | 113 | 23.8 |
| CHEERIOS CEREAL 1 OZ | 2 | 110 | 20 | 4 | 0 | 28.35 | 0.3 |
| CHEESE CRACKERS, PLAIN 10 CRACK | 3 | 50 | 6 | 1 | 6 | 10 | 0.9 |
| CHEESE CRACKERS, SANDWCH,PEANT1 SANDWH | 2 | 40 | 5 | 1 | 1 | 8 | 0.4 |
| CHEESE SAUCE W/ MILK, FRM MIX 1 CUP | 17 | 305 | 23 | 16 | 53 | 279 | 9.3 |
| CHEESEBURGER, 4OZ PATTY 1 SANDWH | 31 | 525 | 40 | 30 | 104 | 194 | 15.1 |
| CHEESEBURGER, REGULAR 1 SANDWH | 15 | 300 | 28 | 15 | 44 | 112 | 7.3 |
| CHEESECAKE 1 CAKE | 213 | 3350 | 317 | 60 | 2053 | 1110 | 119.9 |
| CHEESECAKE 1 PIECE | 18 | 280 | 26 | 5 | 170 | 92 | 9.9 |
| CHERRIES, SOUR,RED,CANND,WATER1 CUP | 0 | 90 | 22 | 2 | 0 | 244 | 0.1 |
| CHERRIES, SWEET, RAW 10 CHERY | 1 | 50 | 11 | 1 | 0 | 68 | 0.1 |
| CHERRY PIE 1 PIE | 107 | 2465 | 363 | 25 | 0 | 945 | 28.4 |
| CHERRY PIE 1 PIECE | 18 | 410 | 61 | 4 | 0 | 158 | 4.7 |
| CHESTNUTS, EUROPEAN, ROASTED 1 CUP | 3 | 350 | 76 | 5 | 0 | 143 | 0.6 |
| CHICKEN A LA KING, HOME RECIPE1 CUP | 34 | 470 | 12 | 27 | 221 | 245 | 12.9 |
| CHICKEN AND NOODLES, HOME RECP1 CUP | 18 | 365 | 26 | 22 | 103 | 240 | 5.1 |
| CHICKEN CHOW MEIN, CANNED 1 CUP | 0 | 95 | 18 | 7 | 8 | 250 | 0.1 |
| CHICKEN CHOW MEIN, HOME RECIPE1 CUP | 10 | 255 | 10 | 31 | 75 | 250 | 4.1 |
| CHICKEN FRANKFURTER 1 FRANK | 9 | 115 | 3 | 6 | 45 | 45 | 2.5 |
| CHICKEN GRAVY FROM DRY MIX 1 CUP | 2 | 85 | 14 | 3 | 3 | 260 | 0.5 |
| CHICKEN GRAVY, CANNED 1 CUP | 14 | 190 | 13 | 5 | 5 | 238 | 3.4 |

| Description of food | Fat (Grams) | Food Energy (calories) | Carbohydrate (Grams) | Protein (Grams) | Cholesterol (Milligrams) | Weight (Grams) | Saturated Fat (Grams) |
|---|---|---|---|---|---|---|---|
| CHICKEN LIVER, COOKED 1 LIVER | 1 | 30 | 0 | 5 | 126 | 20 | 0.4 |
| CHICKEN NOODLE SOUP, CANNED 1 CUP | 2 | 75 | 9 | 4 | 7 | 241 | 0.7 |
| CHICKEN NOODLE SOUP,DEHYD,PRPD1 PKT | 1 | 40 | 6 | 2 | 2 | 188 | 0.2 |
| CHICKEN POTPIE, HOME RECIPE 1 PIECE | 31 | 545 | 42 | 23 | 56 | 232 | 10.3 |
| CHICKEN RICE SOUP, CANNED 1 CUP | 2 | 60 | 7 | 4 | 7 | 241 | 0.5 |
| CHICKEN ROLL, LIGHT 2 SLICES | 4 | 90 | 1 | 11 | 28 | 57 | 1.1 |
| CHICKEN, CANNED, BONELESS 5 OZ | 11 | 235 | 0 | 31 | 88 | 142 | 3.1 |
| CHICKEN, FRIED, BATTER, BREAST4.9 OZ | 18 | 365 | 13 | 35 | 119 | 140 | 4.9 |
| CHICKEN, FRIED, BATTER,DRMSTCK2.5 OZ | 11 | 195 | 6 | 16 | 62 | 72 | 3 |
| CHICKEN, FRIED, FLOUR, BREAST 3.5 OZ | 9 | 220 | 2 | 31 | 87 | 98 | 2.4 |
| CHICKEN, FRIED, FLOUR, DRMSTCK1.7 OZ | 7 | 120 | 1 | 13 | 44 | 49 | 1.8 |
| CHICKEN, ROASTED, BREAST 3.0 OZ | 3 | 140 | 0 | 27 | 73 | 86 | 0.9 |
| CHICKEN, ROASTED, DRUMSTICK 1.6 OZ | 2 | 75 | 0 | 12 | 41 | 44 | 0.7 |
| CHICKEN, STEWED, LIGHT + DARK 1 CUP | 9 | 250 | 0 | 38 | 116 | 140 | 2.6 |
| CHICKPEAS, COOKED, DRAINED 1 CUP | 4 | 270 | 45 | 15 | 0 | 163 | 0.4 |
| CHILI CON CARNE W/ BEANS, CNND1 CUP | 16 | 340 | 31 | 19 | 28 | 255 | 5.8 |
| CHILI POWDER 1 TSP | 0 | 10 | 1 | 0 | 0 | 2.6 | 0.1 |
| CHOCOLATE CHIP COOKIES,COMMRCL4 COOKIE | 9 | 180 | 28 | 2 | 5 | 42 | 2.9 |
| CHOCOLATE CHIP COOKIES,HME RCP4 COOKIE | 11 | 185 | 26 | 2 | 18 | 40 | 3.9 |
| CHOCOLATE CHIP COOKIES,REFRIG 4 COOKIE | 11 | 225 | 32 | 2 | 22 | 48 | 4 |
| CHOCOLATE MILK, LOWFAT 1% 1 CUP | 3 | 160 | 26 | 8 | 7 | 250 | 1.5 |
| CHOCOLATE MILK, LOWFAT 2% 1 CUP | 5 | 180 | 26 | 8 | 17 | 250 | 3.1 |
| CHOCOLATE MILK, REGULAR 1 CUP | 8 | 210 | 26 | 8 | 31 | 250 | 5.3 |
| CHOCOLATE, BITTER OT BAKING 1 OZ | 15 | 145 | 8 | 3 | 0 | 28.35 | 9 |
| CHOP SUEY W/ BEEF + PORK,HMRCP1 CUP | 17 | 300 | 13 | 26 | 68 | 250 | 4.3 |

| Description of food | Fat (Grams) | Food Energy (calories) | Carbohydrate (Grams) | Protein (Grams) | Cholesterol (Milligrams) | Weight (Grams) | Saturated Fat (Grams) |
|---|---|---|---|---|---|---|---|
| CINNAMON 1 TSP | 0 | 5 | 2 | 0 | 0 | 2.3 | 0 |
| CLAM CHOWDER, MANHATTAN, CANND1 CUP | 2 | 80 | 12 | 4 | 2 | 244 | 0.4 |
| CLAM CHOWDER, NEW ENG, W/ MILK1 CUP | 7 | 165 | 17 | 9 | 22 | 248 | 3 |
| CLAMS, CANNED, DRAINED 3 OZ | 2 | 85 | 2 | 13 | 54 | 85 | 0.5 |
| CLAMS, RAW 3 OZ | 1 | 65 | 2 | 11 | 43 | 85 | 0.3 |
| CLUB SODA 12 FL OZ | 0 | 0 | 0 | 0 | 0 | 355 | 0 |
| COCA PWDR W/O NOFAT DRYMLK,PRD1 SERVNG | 9 | 225 | 30 | 9 | 33 | 265 | 5.4 |
| COCA PWDR W/O NONFAT DRY MILK 3/4 OZ | 1 | 75 | 19 | 1 | 0 | 21 | 0.3 |
| COCOA PWDR WITH NONFAT DRYMILK1 OZ | 1 | 100 | 22 | 3 | 1 | 28.35 | 0.6 |
| COCOA PWDR W/ NOFAT DRMLK,PRPD1 SERVNG | 1 | 100 | 22 | 3 | 1 | 206 | 0.6 |
| COCONUT, DRIED, SWEETND,SHREDD1 CUP | 33 | 470 | 44 | 3 | 0 | 93 | 29.3 |
| COCONUT, RAW, PIECE 1 PIECE | 15 | 160 | 7 | 1 | 0 | 45 | 13.4 |
| COCONUT, RAW, SHREDDED 1 CUP | 27 | 285 | 12 | 3 | 0 | 80 | 23.8 |
| COFFEECAKE, CRUMB, FROM MIX 1 CAKE | 41 | 1385 | 225 | 27 | 279 | 430 | 11.8 |
| COFFEECAKE, CRUMB, FROM MIX 1 PIECE | 7 | 230 | 38 | 5 | 47 | 72 | 2 |
| COFFEE, BREWED 6 FL OZ | 0 | 0 | 0 | 0 | 0 | 180 | 0 |
| COFFEE, INSTANT, PREPARED 6 FL OZ | 0 | 0 | 1 | 0 | 0 | 182 | 0 |
| COLA, DIET, ASPARTAME ONLY 12 FL OZ | 0 | 0 | 0 | 0 | 0 | 355 | 0 |
| COLA, DIET, ASPRTAME + SACCHRN12 FL OZ | 0 | 0 | 0 | 0 | 0 | 355 | 0 |
| COLA, DIET, SACCHARIN ONLY 12 FL OZ | 0 | 0 | 0 | 0 | 0 | 355 | 0 |
| COLA, REGULAR 12 FL OZ | 0 | 160 | 41 | 0 | 0 | 369 | 0 |
| COLLARDS, COOKED FROM FROZEN 1 CUP | 1 | 60 | 12 | 5 | 0 | 170 | 0.1 |
| COLLARDS, COOKED FROM RAW 1 CUP | 0 | 25 | 5 | 2 | 0 | 190 | 0.1 |
| COOKED SALAD DRSSING, HOME RCP1 TBSP | 2 | 25 | 2 | 1 | 9 | 16 | 0.5 |
| CORN CHIPS 1 OZ | 9 | 155 | 16 | 2 | 0 | 28.35 | 1.4 |

| Description of food | | Fat (Grams) | Food Energy (calories) | Carbohydrate (Grams) | Protein (Grams) | Cholesterol (Milligrams) | Weight (Grams) | Saturated Fat (Grams) |
|---|---|---|---|---|---|---|---|---|
| CORN FLAKES, KELLOGG'S | 1 OZ | 0 | 110 | 24 | 2 | 0 | 28.35 | 0 |
| CORN FLAKES, TOASTIES | 1 OZ | 0 | 110 | 24 | 2 | 0 | 28.35 | 0 |
| CORN GRITS, COOKED, INSTANT | 1 PKT | 0 | 80 | 18 | 2 | 0 | 137 | 0 |
| CORN GRITS,CKD,REG,WHITE,NOSALT | 1 CUP | 0 | 145 | 31 | 3 | 0 | 242 | 0 |
| CORN GRITS,CKD,REG,WHITE,W/SALT | 1 CUP | 0 | 145 | 31 | 3 | 0 | 242 | 0 |
| CORN GRITS,CKD,REG,YLLW,NOSALT | 1 CUP | 0 | 145 | 31 | 3 | 0 | 242 | 0 |
| CORN GRITS,CKD,REG,YLLW,W/SALT | 1 CUP | 0 | 145 | 31 | 3 | 0 | 242 | 0 |
| CORN MUFFINS, FROM COMMERL MIX | 1 MUFFIN | 6 | 145 | 22 | 3 | 42 | 45 | 1.7 |
| CORN MUFFINS, HOME RECIPE | 1 MUFFIN | 5 | 145 | 21 | 3 | 23 | 45 | 1.5 |
| CORN OIL | 1 CUP | 218 | 1925 | 0 | 0 | 0 | 218 | 27.7 |
| CORN OIL | 1 TBSP | 14 | 125 | 0 | 0 | 0 | 14 | 1.8 |
| CORNMEAL,BOLTED,DRY FORM | 1 CUP | 4 | 440 | 91 | 11 | 0 | 122 | 0.5 |
| CORNMEAL,DEGERMED,ENRICHED,COOK | 1 CUP | 0 | 120 | 26 | 3 | 0 | 240 | 0 |
| CORNMEAL,DEGERMED,ENRICHED,DRY | 1 CUP | 2 | 500 | 108 | 11 | 0 | 138 | 0.2 |
| CORNMEAL,WHOLE-GRND,UNBOLT,DRY | 1 CUP | 5 | 435 | 90 | 11 | 0 | 122 | 0.5 |
| CORN, CNND,CRM STL,WHIT,NO SAL | 1 CUP | 1 | 185 | 46 | 4 | 0 | 256 | 0.2 |
| CORN, CNND,CRM STL,WHIT,W/SALT | 1 CUP | 1 | 185 | 46 | 4 | 0 | 256 | 0.2 |
| CORN, CNND,CRM STL,YLLW,NO SAL | 1 CUP | 1 | 185 | 46 | 4 | 0 | 256 | 0.2 |
| CORN, CNND,CRM STL,YLLW,W/SALT | 1 CUP | 1 | 185 | 46 | 4 | 0 | 256 | 0.2 |
| CORN, COOKED FRM FROZN, WHITE | 1 CUP | 0 | 135 | 34 | 5 | 0 | 165 | 0 |
| CORN, COOKED FRM FROZN, WHITE | 1 EAR | 0 | 60 | 14 | 2 | 0 | 63 | 0.1 |
| CORN, COOKED FRM FROZN, YELLOW | 1 CUP | 0 | 135 | 34 | 5 | 0 | 165 | 0 |
| CORN, COOKED FRM FROZN, YELLOW | 1 EAR | 0 | 60 | 14 | 2 | 0 | 63 | 0.1 |
| CORN, COOKED FROM RAW, WHITE | 1 EAR | 1 | 85 | 19 | 3 | 0 | 77 | 0.2 |
| CORN, COOKED FROM RAW, YELLOW | 1 EAR | 1 | 85 | 19 | 3 | 0 | 77 | 0.2 |

107

| Description of food | Fat (Grams) | Food Energy (calories) | Carbohydrate (Grams) | Protein (Grams) | Cholesterol (Milligrams) | Weight (Grams) | Saturated Fat (Grams) |
|---|---|---|---|---|---|---|---|
| CORN,CNND,WHL KRNL,WHTE,NO SAL1 CUP | 1 | 165 | 41 | 5 | 0 | 210 | 0.2 |
| CORN,CNND,WHL KRNL,WHTE,W/SALT1 CUP | 1 | 165 | 41 | 5 | 0 | 210 | 0.2 |
| CORN,CNND,WHL KRNL,YLLW,NO SAL1 CUP | 1 | 165 | 41 | 5 | 0 | 210 | 0.2 |
| CORN,CNND,WHL KRNL,YLLW,W/SALT1 CUP | 1 | 165 | 41 | 5 | 0 | 210 | 0.2 |
| COTTAGE CHEESE,CREMD,LRGE CURD1 CUP | 10 | 235 | 6 | 28 | 34 | 225 | 6.4 |
| COTTAGE CHEESE,CREMD,SMLL CURD1 CUP | 9 | 215 | 6 | 26 | 31 | 210 | 6 |
| COTTAGE CHEESE,CREMD,W/FRUIT 1 CUP | 8 | 280 | 30 | 22 | 25 | 226 | 4.9 |
| COTTAGE CHEESE,LOWFAT 2% 1 CUP | 4 | 205 | 8 | 31 | 19 | 226 | 2.8 |
| COTTAGE CHEESE,UNCREAMED 1 CUP | 1 | 125 | 3 | 25 | 10 | 145 | 0.4 |
| CR OF CHICKEN SOUP W/ H20,CNND1 CUP | 7 | 115 | 9 | 3 | 10 | 244 | 2.1 |
| CR OF CHICKEN SOUP W/ MLK,CNND1 CUP | 11 | 190 | 15 | 7 | 27 | 248 | 4.6 |
| CR OF MUSHROM SOUP W/ H20,CNND1 CUP | 9 | 130 | 9 | 2 | 2 | 244 | 2.4 |
| CR OF MUSHROM SOUP W/ MLK,CNND1 CUP | 14 | 205 | 15 | 6 | 20 | 248 | 5.1 |
| CRABMEAT, CANNED 1 CUP | 3 | 135 | 1 | 23 | 135 | 135 | 0.5 |
| CRACKED-WHEAT BREAD 1 LOAF | 16 | 1190 | 227 | 42 | 0 | 454 | 3.1 |
| CRACKED-WHEAT BREAD 1 SLICE | 1 | 65 | 12 | 2 | 0 | 25 | 0.2 |
| CRACKED-WHEAT BREAD, TOASTED 1 SLICE | 1 | 65 | 12 | 2 | 0 | 21 | 0.2 |
| CRANBERRY JUICE COCKTAL W/VITC1 CUP | 0 | 145 | 38 | 0 | 0 | 253 | 0 |
| CRANBERRY SAUCE, CANNED,SWTND 1 CUP | 0 | 420 | 108 | 1 | 0 | 277 | 0 |
| CREAM CHEESE 1 OZ | 10 | 100 | 1 | 2 | 31 | 28.35 | 6.2 |
| CREAM OF WHEAT,CKD,MIX N EAT 1 PKT | 0 | 100 | 21 | 3 | 0 | 142 | 0 |
| CREME PIE 1 PIE | 139 | 2710 | 351 | 20 | 46 | 910 | 90.1 |
| CREME PIE 1 PIECE | 23 | 455 | 59 | 3 | 8 | 152 | 15 |
| CRM WHEAT,CKD, QUICK, NO SALT 1 CUP | 0 | 140 | 29 | 4 | 0 | 244 | 0.1 |
| CRM WHEAT,CKD,QUICK, W/ SALT 1 CUP | 0 | 140 | 29 | 4 | 0 | 244 | 0.1 |

| Description of food | Fat (Grams) | Food Energy (calories) | Carbohydrate (Grams) | Protein (Grams) | Cholesterol (Milligrams) | Weight (Grams) | Saturated Fat (Grams) |
|---|---|---|---|---|---|---|---|
| CRM WHEAT,CKD,REG,INST,NO SALT 1 CUP | 0 | 140 | 29 | 4 | 0 | 244 | 0.1 |
| CRM WHEAT,CKD,REG,INST,W/SALT 1 CUP | 0 | 140 | 29 | 4 | 0 | 244 | 0.1 |
| CROISSANTS 1 CROSST | 12 | 235 | 27 | 5 | 13 | 57 | 3.5 |
| CUCUMBER, W/ PEEL 6 SLICES | 0 | 5 | 1 | 0 | 0 | 28 | 0 |
| CURRY POWDER 1 TSP | 0 | 5 | 1 | 0 | 0 | 2 | 0 |
| CUSTARD PIE 1 PIE | 101 | 1985 | 213 | 56 | 1010 | 910 | 33.7 |
| CUSTARD PIE 1 PIECE | 17 | 330 | 36 | 9 | 169 | 152 | 5.6 |
| CUSTARD, BAKED 1 CUP | 15 | 305 | 29 | 14 | 278 | 265 | 6.8 |
| DANDELION GREENS, COOKED, DRND 1 CUP | 1 | 35 | 7 | 2 | 0 | 105 | 0.1 |
| DANISH PASTRY, FRUIT 1 PASTRY | 13 | 235 | 28 | 4 | 56 | 65 | 3.9 |
| DANISH PASTRY, PLAIN, NO NUTS 1 OZ | 6 | 110 | 13 | 2 | 24 | 28.35 | 1.8 |
| DANISH PASTRY, PLAIN, NO NUTS 1 PASTRY | 12 | 220 | 26 | 4 | 49 | 57 | 3.6 |
| DANISH PASTRY, PLAIN, NO NUTS 1 RING | 71 | 1305 | 152 | 21 | 292 | 340 | 21.8 |
| DATES 10 DATES | 0 | 230 | 61 | 2 | 0 | 83 | 0.1 |
| DATES, CHOPPED 1 CUP | 1 | 490 | 131 | 4 | 0 | 178 | 0.3 |
| DEVIL'S FOOD CAKE,CHOCFRST,FMX 1 CAKE | 136 | 3755 | 645 | 49 | 598 | 1107 | 55.6 |
| DEVIL'S FOOD CAKE,CHOCFRST,FMX 1 CUPCAK | 4 | 120 | 20 | 2 | 19 | 35 | 1.8 |
| DEVIL'S FOOD CAKE,CHOCFRST,FMX 1 PIECE | 8 | 235 | 40 | 3 | 37 | 69 | 3.5 |
| DOUGHNUTS, CAKE TYPE, PLAIN 1 DONUT | 12 | 210 | 24 | 3 | 20 | 50 | 2.8 |
| DOUGHNUTS, YEAST-LEAVEND,GLZED 1 DONUT | 13 | 235 | 26 | 4 | 21 | 60 | 5.2 |
| DUCK, ROASTED, FLESH ONLY 1/2 DUCK | 25 | 445 | 0 | 52 | 197 | 221 | 9.2 |
| EGGNOG 1 CUP | 19 | 340 | 34 | 10 | 149 | 254 | 11.3 |
| EGGPLANT, COOKED, STEAMED 1 CUP | 0 | 25 | 6 | 1 | 0 | 96 | 0 |
| EGGS, COOKED, FRIED 1 EGG | 7 | 90 | 1 | 6 | 211 | 46 | 1.9 |
| EGGS, COOKED, HARD-COOKED 1 EGG | 5 | 75 | 1 | 6 | 213 | 50 | 1.6 |

| Description of food | Fat (Grams) | Food Energy (calories) | Carbohydrate (Grams) | Protein (Grams) | Cholesterol (Milligrams) | Weight (Grams) | Saturated Fat (Grams) |
|---|---|---|---|---|---|---|---|
| EGGS, COOKED, POACHED 1 EGG | 5 | 75 | 1 | 6 | 212 | 50 | 1.5 |
| EGGS, COOKED, SCRAMBLED/OMELET 1 EGG | 7 | 100 | 1 | 7 | 215 | 61 | 2.2 |
| EGGS, RAW, WHITE 1 WHITE | 0 | 15 | 0 | 4 | 0 | 33 | 0 |
| EGGS, RAW, WHOLE 1 EGG | 5 | 75 | 1 | 6 | 213 | 50 | 1.6 |
| EGGS, RAW, YOLK 1 YOLK | 5 | 60 | 0 | 3 | 213 | 17 | 1.6 |
| ENCHILADA 1 ENCHLD | 16 | 235 | 24 | 20 | 19 | 230 | 7.7 |
| ENDIVE, CURLY, RAW 1 CUP | 0 | 10 | 2 | 1 | 0 | 50 | 0 |
| ENG MUFFIN, EGG, CHEESE, BACON 1 SANDWH | 18 | 360 | 31 | 18 | 213 | 138 | 8 |
| ENGLISH MUFFINS, PLAIN 1 MUFFIN | 1 | 140 | 27 | 5 | 0 | 57 | 0.3 |
| ENGLISH MUFFINS, PLAIN, TOASTD 1 MUFFIN | 1 | 140 | 27 | 5 | 0 | 50 | 0.3 |
| EVAPORATED MILK, SKIM, CANNED 1 CUP | 1 | 200 | 29 | 19 | 9 | 255 | 0.3 |
| EVAPORATED MILK, WHOLE, CANNED 1 CUP | 19 | 340 | 25 | 17 | 74 | 252 | 11.6 |
| FATS, COOKING/VEGETBL SHORTENG 1 CUP | 205 | 1810 | 0 | 0 | 0 | 205 | 51.3 |
| FATS, COOKING/VEGETBL SHORTENG 1 TBSP | 13 | 115 | 0 | 0 | 0 | 13 | 3.3 |
| FETA CHEESE 1 OZ | 6 | 75 | 1 | 4 | 25 | 28.35 | 4.2 |
| FIG BARS 4 COOKIE | 4 | 210 | 42 | 2 | 27 | 56 | 1 |
| FIGS, DRIED 10 FIGS | 2 | 475 | 122 | 6 | 0 | 187 | 0.4 |
| FILBERTS, (HAZELNUTS) CHOPPED 1 CUP | 72 | 725 | 18 | 15 | 0 | 115 | 5.3 |
| FILBERTS, (HAZELNUTS) CHOPPED 1 OZ | 18 | 180 | 4 | 4 | 0 | 28.35 | 1.3 |
| FISH SANDWICH, LGE, W/O CHEESE 1 SANDWH | 27 | 470 | 41 | 18 | 91 | 170 | 6.3 |
| FISH SANDWICH, REG, W/ CHEESE 1 SANDWH | 23 | 420 | 39 | 16 | 56 | 140 | 6.3 |
| FISH STICKS, FROZEN, REHEATED 1 STICK | 3 | 70 | 4 | 6 | 26 | 28 | 0.8 |
| FLOUNDER OR SOLE, BAKED, BUTTR 3 OZ | 6 | 120 | 0 | 16 | 68 | 85 | 3.2 |
| FLOUNDER OR SOLE, BAKED, MARGRN 3 OZ | 6 | 120 | 0 | 16 | 55 | 85 | 1.2 |
| FLOUNDER OR SOLE, BAKED, W/OFAT 3 OZ | 1 | 80 | 0 | 17 | 59 | 85 | 0.3 |

| Description of food | | Fat (Grams) | Food Energy (calories) | Carbohydrate (Grams) | Protein (Grams) | Cholesterol (Milligrams) | Weight (Grams) | Saturated Fat (Grams) |
|---|---|---|---|---|---|---|---|---|
| FONDANT, UNCOATED | 1 OZ | 0 | 105 | 27 | 0 | 0 | 28.35 | 0 |
| FRANKFURTER, COOKED | 1 FRANK | 13 | 145 | 1 | 5 | 23 | 45 | 4.8 |
| FRENCH BREAD | 1 SLICE | 1 | 100 | 18 | 3 | 0 | 35 | 0.3 |
| FRENCH OR VIENNA BREAD | 1 LOAF | 18 | 1270 | 230 | 43 | 0 | 454 | 3.8 |
| FRENCH SALAD DRESSING, LOCALORI | TBSP | 2 | 25 | 2 | 0 | 0 | 16 | 0.2 |
| FRENCH SALAD DRESSING, REGULAR1 | TBSP | 9 | 85 | 1 | 0 | 0 | 16 | 1.4 |
| FRENCH TOAST, HOME RECIPE | 1 SLICE | 7 | 155 | 17 | 6 | 112 | 65 | 1.6 |
| FRIED PIE, APPLE | 1 PIE | 14 | 255 | 31 | 2 | 14 | 85 | 5.8 |
| FRIED PIE, CHERRY | 1 PIE | 14 | 250 | 32 | 2 | 13 | 85 | 5.8 |
| FROOT LOOPS CEREAL | 1 OZ | 1 | 110 | 25 | 2 | 0 | 28.35 | 0.2 |
| FRUIT COCKTAIL,CNND,HEAVYSYRUP1 | CUP | 0 | 185 | 48 | 1 | 0 | 255 | 0 |
| FRUIT COCKTAIL,CNND,JUICE PACK1 | CUP | 0 | 115 | 29 | 1 | 0 | 248 | 0 |
| FRUIT PUNCH DRINK, CANNED | 6 FL OZ | 0 | 85 | 22 | 0 | 0 | 190 | 0 |
| FRUITCAKE,DARK, FROM HOMERRCIP1 | CAKE | 228 | 5185 | 783 | 74 | 640 | 1361 | 47.6 |
| FRUITCAKE,DARK, FROM HOMERECIP1 | PIECE | 7 | 165 | 25 | 2 | 20 | 43 | 1.5 |
| FUDGE, CHOCOLATE, PLAIN | 1 OZ | 3 | 115 | 21 | 1 | 1 | 28.35 | 2.1 |
| GARLIC POWDER | 1 TSP | 0 | 10 | 2 | 0 | 0 | 2.8 | 0 |
| GELATIN DESSERT, PREPARED | 1/2 CUP | 0 | 70 | 17 | 2 | 0 | 120 | 0 |
| GELATIN, DRY | 1 ENVELP | 0 | 25 | 0 | 6 | 0 | 7 | 0 |
| GINGER ALE | 12 FL OZ | 0 | 125 | 32 | 0 | 0 | 366 | 0 |
| GINGERBREAD CAKE, FROM MIX | 1 CAKE | 39 | 1575 | 291 | 18 | 6 | 570 | 9.6 |
| GINGERBREAD CAKE, FROM MIX | 1 PIECE | 4 | 175 | 32 | 2 | 1 | 63 | 1.1 |
| GIN,RUM,VODKA,WHISKY 80-PROOF | 1.5 F OZ | 0 | 95 | 0 | 0 | 0 | 42 | 0 |
| GIN,RUM,VODKA,WHISKY 86-PROOF | 1.5 F OZ | 0 | 105 | 0 | 0 | 0 | 42 | 0 |
| GIN,RUM,VODKA,WHISKY 90-PROOF | 1.5 F OZ | 0 | 110 | 0 | 0 | 0 | 42 | 0 |

111

| Description of food | | Fat (Grams) | Food Energy (calories) | Carbohydrate (Grams) | Protein (Grams) | Cholesterol (Milligrams) | Weight (Grams) | Saturated Fat (Grams) |
|---|---|---|---|---|---|---|---|---|
| GOLDEN GRAHAMS CEREAL | 1 OZ | 1 | 110 | 24 | 2 | 0 | 28.35 | 0.7 |
| GRAHAM CRACKER, PLAIN | 2 CRACKR | 1 | 60 | 11 | 1 | 0 | 14 | 0.4 |
| GRAPE-NUTS CEREAL | 1 OZ | 0 | 100 | 23 | 3 | 0 | 28.35 | 0 |
| GRAPE DRINK, CANNED | 6 FL OZ | 0 | 100 | 26 | 0 | 0 | 187 | 0 |
| GRAPE JUICE, CANNED | 1 CUP | 0 | 155 | 38 | 1 | 0 | 253 | 0.1 |
| GRAPE SODA | 12 FL OZ | 0 | 180 | 46 | 0 | 0 | 372 | 0 |
| GRAPEFRT JCE,CNCN,UNSWTEN | 6 FL OZ | 1 | 300 | 72 | 4 | 0 | 207 | 0.1 |
| GRAPEFRT JCE,FRZN,DLTD,UNSWTEN | 1 CUP | 0 | 100 | 24 | 1 | 0 | 247 | 0 |
| GRAPEFRUIT JUICE, CANNED,SWTND | 1 CUP | 0 | 115 | 28 | 1 | 0 | 250 | 0 |
| GRAPEFRUIT JUICE, CANNED,UNSWT | 1 CUP | 0 | 95 | 22 | 1 | 0 | 247 | 0 |
| GRAPEFRUIT JUICE, RAW | 1 CUP | 0 | 95 | 23 | 1 | 0 | 247 | 0 |
| GRAPEFRUIT, CANNED, SYRUP PACK | 1 CUP | 0 | 150 | 39 | 1 | 0 | 254 | 0 |
| GRAPEFRUIT, RAW, PINK | 1/2 FRUT | 0 | 40 | 10 | 1 | 0 | 120 | 0 |
| GRAPEFRUIT, RAW, WHITE | 1/2 FRUT | 0 | 40 | 10 | 1 | 0 | 120 | 0 |
| GRAPEJCE,FRZN,CONCEN,SWTND,W/C | 6 FL OZ | 1 | 385 | 96 | 1 | 0 | 216 | 0.2 |
| GRAPEJCE,FRZN,DILUTD,SWTND,W/C | 1 CUP | 0 | 125 | 32 | 0 | 0 | 250 | 0.1 |
| GRAPES, EUROPEAN, RAW, THOMPSN | 10 GRAPE | 0 | 35 | 9 | 0 | 0 | 50 | 0.1 |
| GRAPES, EUROPEAN, RAW, TOKAY | 10 GRAPE | 0 | 40 | 10 | 0 | 0 | 57 | 0.1 |
| GRAVY AND TURKEY, FROZEN | 5 OZ | 4 | 95 | 7 | 8 | 26 | 142 | 1.2 |
| GREAT NORTHN BEANS,DRY,CKD,DRN | 1 CUP | 1 | 210 | 38 | 14 | 0 | 180 | 0.1 |
| GROUND BEEF, BROILED, LEAN | 3 OZ | 16 | 230 | 0 | 21 | 74 | 85 | 6.2 |
| GROUND BEEF, BROILED, REGULAR | 3 OZ | 18 | 245 | 0 | 20 | 76 | 85 | 6.9 |
| GUM DROPS | 1 OZ | 0 | 100 | 25 | 0 | 0 | 28.35 | 0 |
| HADDOCK, BREADED, FRIED | 3 OZ | 9 | 175 | 7 | 17 | 75 | 85 | 2.4 |
| HALF AND HALF, CREAM | 1 CUP | 28 | 315 | 10 | 7 | 89 | 242 | 17.3 |

| Description of food | Fat (Grams) | Food Energy (calories) | Carbohydrate (Grams) | Protein (Grams) | Cholesterol (Milligrams) | Weight (Grams) | Saturated Fat (Grams) |
|---|---|---|---|---|---|---|---|
| HALF AND HALF, CREAM 1 TBSP | 2 | 20 | 1 | 0 | 6 | 15 | 1.1 |
| HALIBUT, BROILED, BUTTER,LEMJU3 OZ | 6 | 140 | 0 | 20 | 62 | 85 | 3.3 |
| HAMBURGER, 4OZ PATTY 1 SANDWH | 21 | 445 | 38 | 25 | 71 | 174 | 7.1 |
| HAMBURGER, REGULAR 1 SANDWH | 11 | 245 | 28 | 12 | 32 | 98 | 4.4 |
| HARD CANDY 1 OZ | 0 | 110 | 28 | 0 | 0 | 28.35 | 0 |
| HERRING, PICKLED 3 OZ | 13 | 190 | 0 | 17 | 85 | 85 | 4.3 |
| HOLLANDAISE SCE, W/ H2O,FRM MX1 CUP | 20 | 240 | 14 | 5 | 52 | 259 | 11.6 |
| HONEY 1 CUP | 0 | 1030 | 279 | 1 | 0 | 339 | 0 |
| HONEY 1 TBSP | 0 | 65 | 17 | 0 | 0 | 21 | 0 |
| HONEY NUT CHEERIOS CEREAL 1 OZ | 1 | 105 | 23 | 3 | 0 | 28.35 | 0.1 |
| HONEYDEW MELON, RAW 1/10 MEL | 0 | 45 | 12 | 1 | 0 | 129 | 0 |
| ICE CREAM, VANILLA, REGULR 11% 1 CUP | 14 | 270 | 32 | 5 | 59 | 133 | 8.9 |
| ICE CREAM, VANILLA, REGULR 11% 1/2 GALN | 115 | 2155 | 254 | 38 | 476 | 1064 | 71.3 |
| ICE CREAM, VANILLA, REGULR 11% 3 FL OZ | 5 | 100 | 12 | 2 | 22 | 50 | 3.4 |
| ICE CREAM, VANILLA, RICH 16% FT1 CUP | 24 | 350 | 32 | 4 | 88 | 148 | 14.7 |
| ICE CREAM, VANILLA, RICH 16% FT1/2 GAL | 190 | 2805 | 256 | 33 | 703 | 1188 | 118.3 |
| ICE CREAM, VANILLA, SOFT SERVE 1 CUP | 23 | 375 | 38 | 7 | 153 | 173 | 13.5 |
| ICE MILK, VANILLA, 4% FAT 1 CUP | 6 | 185 | 29 | 5 | 18 | 131 | 3.5 |
| ICE MILK, VANILLA, 4% FAT 1/2 GAL | 45 | 1470 | 232 | 41 | 146 | 1048 | 28.1 |
| ICE MILK, VANILLA,SOFTSERV 3% 1 CUP | 5 | 225 | 38 | 8 | 13 | 175 | 2.9 |
| IMITATION CREAMERS, LIQUID FRZ1 TBSP | 1 | 20 | 2 | 0 | 0 | 15 | 1.4 |
| IMITATION CREAMERS, POWDERED 1 TSP | 1 | 10 | 1 | 0 | 0 | 2 | 0.7 |
| IMITATION WHIPPED TOPPING,FRZN1 CUP | 19 | 240 | 17 | 1 | 0 | 75 | 16.3 |
| IMITATION WHIPPED TOPPING,FRZN1 TBSP | 1 | 15 | 1 | 0 | 0 | 4 | 0.9 |
| IMITATN SOUR DRESSING 1 CUP | 39 | 415 | 11 | 8 | 13 | 235 | 31.2 |

| Description of food | Fat (Grams) | Food Energy (calories) | Carbohydrate (Grams) | Protein (Grams) | Cholesterol (Milligrams) | Weight (Grams) | Saturated Fat (Grams) |
|---|---|---|---|---|---|---|---|
| IMITATN SOUR DRESSING 1 TBSP | 2 | 20 | 1 | 0 | 1 | 12 | 1.6 |
| IMITATN WHIPD TOPING,PRESSRZD 1 CUP | 16 | 185 | 11 | 1 | 0 | 70 | 13.2 |
| IMITATN WHIPD TOPING,PRESSRZD 1 TBSP | 1 | 10 | 1 | 0 | 0 | 4 | 0.8 |
| IMITATN WHIPD TOPING,PWDRD,PRP1 CUP | 10 | 150 | 13 | 3 | 8 | 80 | 8.5 |
| IMITATN WHIPD TOPING,PWDRD,PRP1 TBSP | 0 | 10 | 1 | 0 | 0 | 4 | 0.4 |
| ITALIAN BREAD 1 LOAF | 4 | 1255 | 256 | 41 | 0 | 454 | 0.6 |
| ITALIAN BREAD 1 SLICE | 0 | 85 | 17 | 3 | 0 | 30 | 0 |
| ITALIAN SALAD DRESSING,LOCALOR1 TBSP | 0 | 5 | 2 | 0 | 0 | 15 | 0 |
| ITALIAN SALAD DRESSING,REGULAR1 TBSP | 9 | 80 | 1 | 0 | 0 | 15 | 1.3 |
| JAMS AND PRESERVES 1 PKT | 0 | 40 | 10 | 0 | 0 | 14 | 0 |
| JAMS AND PRESERVES 1 TBSP | 0 | 55 | 14 | 0 | 0 | 20 | 0 |
| JELLIES 1 PKT | 0 | 40 | 10 | 0 | 0 | 14 | 0 |
| JELLIES 1 TBSP | 0 | 50 | 13 | 0 | 0 | 18 | 0 |
| JELLY BEANS 1 OZ | 0 | 105 | 26 | 0 | 0 | 28.35 | 0 |
| JERUSALEM-ARTICHOKE, RAW 1 CUP | 0 | 115 | 26 | 3 | 0 | 150 | 0 |
| KALE, COOKED FROM FROZEN 1 CUP | 1 | 40 | 7 | 4 | 0 | 130 | 0.1 |
| KALE, COOKED FROM RAW 1 CUP | 1 | 40 | 7 | 2 | 0 | 130 | 0.1 |
| KIWIFRUIT, RAW 1 KIWI | 0 | 45 | 11 | 1 | 0 | 76 | 0 |
| KOHLRABI, COOKED, DRAINED 1 CUP | 0 | 50 | 11 | 3 | 0 | 165 | 0 |
| LAMB, RIB, ROASTED, LEAN ONLY 2 OZ | 7 | 130 | 0 | 15 | 50 | 57 | 3.2 |
| LAMB, RIB, ROASTED, LEAN + FAT3 OZ | 26 | 315 | 0 | 18 | 77 | 85 | 12.1 |
| LAMB,CHOPS,ARM,BRAISED,LEAN 1.7 OZ | 7 | 135 | 0 | 17 | 59 | 48 | 2.9 |
| LAMB,CHOPS,ARM,BRAISED,LEAN+FT2.2 OZ | 15 | 220 | 0 | 20 | 77 | 63 | 6.9 |
| LAMB,CHOPS,LOIN,BROIL,LEAN 2.3 OZ | 6 | 140 | 0 | 19 | 60 | 64 | 2.6 |
| LAMB,CHOPS,LOIN,BROIL,LEAN+FAT2.8 OZ | 16 | 235 | 0 | 22 | 78 | 80 | 7.3 |

| Description of food | | Fat (Grams) | Food Energy (calories) | Carbohydrate (Grams) | Protein (Grams) | Cholesterol (Milligrams) | Weight (Grams) | Saturated Fat (Grams) |
|---|---|---|---|---|---|---|---|---|
| LAMB,LEG,ROASTED, LEAN ONLY | 2.6 OZ | 6 | 140 | 0 | 20 | 65 | 73 | 2.4 |
| LAMB,LEG,ROASTED, LEAN+ FAT | 3 OZ | 13 | 205 | 0 | 22 | 78 | 85 | 5.6 |
| LARD | 1 CUP | 205 | 1850 | 0 | 0 | 195 | 205 | 80.4 |
| LARD | 1 TBSP | 13 | 115 | 0 | 0 | 12 | 13 | 5.1 |
| LEMON-LIME SODA | 12 FL OZ | 0 | 155 | 39 | 0 | 0 | 372 | 0 |
| LEMON JUICE, CANNED | 1 CUP | 1 | 50 | 16 | 1 | 0 | 244 | 0.1 |
| LEMON JUICE, CANNED | 1 TBSP | 0 | 5 | 1 | 0 | 0 | 15 | 0 |
| LEMON JUICE, RAW | 1 CUP | 0 | 60 | 21 | 1 | 0 | 244 | 0 |
| LEMON JUICE,FRZN,SINGLE-STRNGH | 6 FL OZ | 1 | 55 | 16 | 1 | 0 | 244 | 0.1 |
| LEMON MERINGUE PIE | 1 PIE | 86 | 2140 | 317 | 31 | 857 | 840 | 26 |
| LEMON MERINGUE PIE | 1 PIECE | 14 | 355 | 53 | 5 | 143 | 140 | 4.3 |
| LEMONADE,CONCENTRATE,FRZ,UNDIL | 6 FL OZ | 0 | 425 | 112 | 0 | 0 | 219 | 0 |
| LEMONADE,CONCEN,FRZEN,DILUTED | 6 FL OZ | 0 | 80 | 21 | 0 | 0 | 185 | 0 |
| LEMONS, RAW | 1 LEMON | 0 | 15 | 5 | 1 | 0 | 58 | 0 |
| LENTILS, DRY, COOKED | 1 CUP | 1 | 215 | 38 | 16 | 0 | 200 | 0.1 |
| LETTUCE, BUTTERHEAD, RAW,HEAD | 1 HEAD | 0 | 20 | 4 | 2 | 0 | 163 | 0 |
| LETTUCE, BUTTERHEAD, RAW,LEAVE | 1 LEAF | 0 | 0 | 0 | 0 | 0 | 15 | 0 |
| LETTUCE, CRISPHEAD, RAW, HEAD | 1 HEAD | 1 | 70 | 11 | 5 | 0 | 539 | 0.1 |
| LETTUCE, CRISPHEAD, RAW,PIECES | 1 CUP | 0 | 5 | 1 | 1 | 0 | 55 | 0 |
| LETTUCE, CRISPHEAD, RAW,WEDGE | 1 WEDGE | 0 | 20 | 3 | 1 | 0 | 135 | 0 |
| LETTUCE, LOOSELEAF | 1 CUP | 0 | 10 | 2 | 1 | 0 | 56 | 0 |
| LIGHT, COFFEE OR TABLE CREAM | 1 CUP | 46 | 470 | 9 | 6 | 159 | 240 | 28.8 |
| LIGHT, COFFEE OR TABLE CREAM | 1 TBSP | 3 | 30 | 1 | 0 | 10 | 15 | 1.8 |
| LIMA BEANS, DRY, COOKED,DRANED | 1 CUP | 1 | 260 | 49 | 16 | 0 | 190 | 0.2 |
| LIMA BEANS,BABY, FRZN,CKED,DRN | 1 CUP | 1 | 190 | 35 | 12 | 0 | 180 | 0.1 |

| Description of food | Fat (Grams) | Food Energy (calories) | Carbohydrate (Grams) | Protein (Grams) | Cholesterol (Milligrams) | Weight (Grams) | Saturated Fat (Grams) |
|---|---|---|---|---|---|---|---|
| LIMA BEANS,THICK SEED,FRZN,CKD1 CUP | 1 | 170 | 32 | 10 | 0 | 170 | 0.1 |
| LIME JUICE, RAW 1 CUP | 0 | 65 | 22 | 1 | 0 | 246 | 0 |
| LIME JUICE,CANNED 1 CUP | 1 | 50 | 16 | 1 | 0 | 246 | 0.1 |
| LIMEADE,CONCENTRATE,FRZN,UNDIL6 FL OZ | 0 | 410 | 108 | 0 | 0 | 218 | 0 |
| LIMEADE,CONCEN,FROZEN,DILUTED 6 FL OZ | 0 | 75 | 20 | 0 | 0 | 185 | 0 |
| LUCKY CHARMS CEREAL 1 OZ | 1 | 110 | 23 | 3 | 0 | 28.35 | 0.2 |
| MACADAMIA NUTS, OILRSTD,SALTED1 CUP | 103 | 960 | 17 | 10 | 0 | 134 | 15.4 |
| MACADAMIA NUTS, OILRSTD,SALTED1 OZ | 22 | 205 | 4 | 2 | 0 | 28.35 | 3.2 |
| MACADAMIA NUTS, OILRSTD,UNSALT1 CUP | 103 | 960 | 17 | 10 | 0 | 134 | 15.4 |
| MACADAMIA NUTS, OILRSTD,UNSALT1 OZ | 22 | 205 | 4 | 2 | 0 | 28.35 | 3.2 |
| MACARONI AND CHEESE, CANNED 1 CUP | 10 | 230 | 26 | 9 | 24 | 240 | 4.7 |
| MACARONI AND CHEESE, HOME RCPE1 CUP | 22 | 430 | 40 | 17 | 44 | 200 | 9.8 |
| MACARONI, COOKED, FIRM 1 CUP | 1 | 190 | 39 | 7 | 0 | 130 | 0.1 |
| MACARONI, COOKED, TENDER, HOT 1 CUP | 1 | 155 | 32 | 5 | 0 | 140 | 0.1 |
| MACARONI, COOKED, TENDER,COLD 1 CUP | 0 | 115 | 24 | 4 | 0 | 105 | 0.1 |
| MALT-O-MEAL, WITH SALT 1 CUP | 0 | 120 | 26 | 4 | 0 | 240 | 0 |
| MALT-O-MEAL, W/O SALT 1 CUP | 0 | 120 | 26 | 4 | 0 | 240 | 0 |
| MALTED MILK, CHOCOLATE, POWDER3/4 OZ | 1 | 85 | 18 | 1 | 1 | 21 | 0.5 |
| MALTED MILK,CHOCOLATE, PWDRPPD1 SERVNG | 9 | 235 | 29 | 9 | 34 | 265 | 5.5 |
| MALTED MILK,NATURAL, POWDER 3/4 OZ | 2 | 85 | 15 | 3 | 4 | 21 | 0.9 |
| MALTED MILK,NATURAL, PWDR PPRD1 SERVNG | 10 | 235 | 27 | 11 | 37 | 265 | 6 |
| MANGOS, RAW 1 MANGO | 1 | 135 | 35 | 1 | 0 | 207 | 0.1 |
| MARGARINE, IMITATION 40% FAT 1 TBSP | 5 | 50 | 0 | 0 | 0 | 14 | 1.1 |
| MARGARINE, IMITATION 40% FAT 8 OZ | 88 | 785 | 1 | 1 | 0 | 227 | 17.5 |
| MARGARINE, REGULR,HARD,80% FAT1 PAT | 4 | 35 | 0 | 0 | 0 | 5 | 0.8 |

| Description of food | Fat (Grams) | Food Energy (calories) | Carbohydrate (Grams) | Protein (Grams) | Cholesterol (Milligrams) | Weight (Grams) | Saturated Fat (Grams) |
|---|---|---|---|---|---|---|---|
| MARGARINE, REGULR,HARD,80% FAT 1 TBSP | 11 | 100 | 0 | 0 | 0 | 14 | 2.2 |
| MARGARINE, REGULR,HARD,80% FAT 1/2 CUP | 91 | 810 | 1 | 1 | 0 | 113 | 17.9 |
| MARGARINE, REGULR,SOFT,80% FAT 1 TBSP | 11 | 100 | 0 | 0 | 0 | 14 | 1.9 |
| MARGARINE, REGULR,SOFT,80% FAT 8 OZ | 183 | 1625 | 1 | 2 | 0 | 227 | 31.3 |
| MARGARINE, SPREAD,HARD,60% FAT 1 PAT | 3 | 25 | 0 | 0 | 0 | 5 | 0.7 |
| MARGARINE, SPREAD,HARD,60% FAT 1 TBSP | 9 | 75 | 0 | 0 | 0 | 14 | 2 |
| MARGARINE, SPREAD,HARD,60% FAT 1/2 CUP | 69 | 610 | 0 | 1 | 0 | 113 | 15.9 |
| MARGARINE, SPREAD,SOFT,60% FAT 1 TBSP | 9 | 75 | 0 | 0 | 0 | 14 | 1.8 |
| MARGARINE, SPREAD,SOFT,60% FAT 8 OZ | 138 | 1225 | 0 | 1 | 0 | 227 | 29.1 |
| MARSHMALLOWS 1 OZ | 0 | 90 | 23 | 1 | 0 | 28.35 | 0 |
| MAYONNAISE TYPE SALAD DRESSING 1 TBSP | 5 | 60 | 4 | 0 | 4 | 15 | 0.7 |
| MAYONNAISE, IMITATION 1 TBSP | 3 | 35 | 2 | 0 | 4 | 15 | 0.5 |
| MAYONNAISE, REGULAR 1 TBSP | 11 | 100 | 0 | 0 | 8 | 14 | 1.7 |
| MELBA TOAST, PLAIN 1 PIECE | 0 | 20 | 4 | 1 | 0 | 5 | 0.1 |
| MILK CHOCOLATE CANDY, PLAIN 1 OZ | 9 | 145 | 16 | 2 | 6 | 28.35 | 5.4 |
| MILK CHOCOLATE CANDY,W/ ALMOND 1 OZ | 10 | 150 | 15 | 3 | 5 | 28.35 | 4.8 |
| MILK CHOCOLATE CANDY,W/ PENUTS 1 OZ | 11 | 155 | 13 | 4 | 5 | 28.35 | 4.2 |
| MILK CHOCOLATE CANDY,W/ RICE C 1 OZ | 7 | 140 | 18 | 2 | 6 | 28.35 | 4.4 |
| MILK, LOFAT, 1%, ADDED SOLIDS 1 CUP | 2 | 105 | 12 | 9 | 10 | 245 | 1.5 |
| MILK, LOFAT, 1%, NO ADDEDSOLID 1 CUP | 3 | 100 | 12 | 8 | 10 | 244 | 1.6 |
| MILK, LOFAT, 2%, ADDED SOLIDS 1 CUP | 5 | 125 | 12 | 9 | 18 | 245 | 2.9 |
| MILK, LOFAT, 2%, NO ADDEDSOLID 1 CUP | 5 | 120 | 12 | 8 | 18 | 244 | 2.9 |
| MILK, SKIM, ADDED MILK SOLIDS 1 CUP | 1 | 90 | 12 | 9 | 5 | 245 | 0.4 |
| MILK, SKIM, NO ADDED MILKSOLID 1 CUP | 0 | 85 | 12 | 8 | 4 | 245 | 0.3 |
| MILK, WHOLE, 3.3% FAT 1 CUP | 8 | 150 | 11 | 8 | 33 | 244 | 5.1 |

| Description of food | | Fat (Grams) | Food Energy (calories) | Carbohydrate (Grams) | Protein (Grams) | Cholesterol (Milligrams) | Weight (Grams) | Saturated Fat (Grams) |
|---|---|---|---|---|---|---|---|---|
| MINESTRONE SOUP, CANNED | 1 CUP | 3 | 80 | 11 | 4 | 2 | 241 | 0.6 |
| MISO | 1 CUP | 13 | 470 | 65 | 29 | 0 | 276 | 1.8 |
| MIXED GRAIN BREAD | 1 LOAF | 17 | 1165 | 212 | 45 | 0 | 454 | 3.2 |
| MIXED GRAIN BREAD | 1 SLICE | 1 | 65 | 12 | 2 | 0 | 25 | 0.2 |
| MIXED GRAIN BREAD, TOASTED | 1 SLICE | 1 | 65 | 12 | 2 | 0 | 23 | 0.2 |
| MIXED NUTS W/ PEANTS,DRY,SALTD | 1 OZ | 15 | 170 | 7 | 5 | 0 | 28.35 | 2 |
| MIXED NUTS W/ PEANTS,DRY,UNSLT | 1 OZ | 15 | 170 | 7 | 5 | 0 | 28.35 | 2 |
| MIXED NUTS W/ PEANTS,OIL,SALTD | 1 OZ | 16 | 175 | 6 | 5 | 0 | 28.35 | 2.5 |
| MIXED NUTS W/ PEANTS,OIL,UNSLT | 1 OZ | 16 | 175 | 6 | 5 | 0 | 28.35 | 2.5 |
| MOLASSES, CANE, BLACKSTRAP | 2 TBSP | 0 | 85 | 22 | 0 | 0 | 40 | 0 |
| MOZZARELLA CHEESE, WHOLE MILK | 1 OZ | 6 | 80 | 1 | 6 | 22 | 28.35 | 3.7 |
| MOZZARELLA CHESE,SKIM, LOMOIST | 1 OZ | 5 | 80 | 1 | 8 | 15 | 28.35 | 3.1 |
| MUENSTER CHEESE | 1 OZ | 9 | 105 | 0 | 7 | 27 | 28.35 | 5.4 |
| MUSHROOM GRAVY, CANNED | 1 CUP | 6 | 120 | 13 | 3 | 0 | 238 | 1 |
| MUSHROOMS, CANNED, DRND,W/SALT | 1 CUP | 0 | 35 | 8 | 3 | 0 | 156 | 0.1 |
| MUSHROOMS, COOKED, DRAINED | 1 CUP | 1 | 40 | 8 | 3 | 0 | 156 | 0.1 |
| MUSHROOMS, RAW | 1 CUP | 0 | 20 | 3 | 1 | 0 | 70 | 0 |
| MUSTARD GREENS, COOKED, DRANED | 1 CUP | 0 | 20 | 3 | 3 | 0 | 140 | 0 |
| MUSTARD, PREPARED, YELLOW | 1 TSP | 0 | 5 | 0 | 0 | 0 | 5 | 0 |
| NATURE VALLEY GRANOLA CEREAL | 1 OZ | 5 | 125 | 19 | 3 | 0 | 28.35 | 3.3 |
| NECTARINES, RAW | 1 NECTRN | 1 | 65 | 16 | 1 | 0 | 136 | 0.1 |
| NONFAT DRY MILK, INSTANTIZED | 1 CUP | 0 | 245 | 35 | 24 | 12 | 68 | 0.3 |
| NONFAT DRY MILK, INSTANTIZED | 1 ENVLPE | 1 | 325 | 47 | 32 | 17 | 91 | 0.4 |
| NOODLES, CHOW MEIN, CANNED | 1 CUP | 11 | 220 | 26 | 6 | 5 | 45 | 2.1 |
| NOODLES, EGG, COOKED | 1 CUP | 2 | 200 | 37 | 7 | 50 | 160 | 0.5 |

| Description of food | | Fat (Grams) | Food Energy (calories) | Carbohydrate (Grams) | Protein (Grams) | Cholesterol (Milligrams) | Weight (Grams) | Saturated Fat (Grams) |
|---|---|---|---|---|---|---|---|---|
| OATMEAL BREAD | 1 LOAF | 20 | 1145 | 212 | 38 | 0 | 454 | 3.7 |
| OATMEAL BREAD | 1 SLICE | 1 | 65 | 12 | 2 | 0 | 25 | 0.2 |
| OATMEAL BREAD, TOASTED | 1 SLICE | 1 | 65 | 12 | 2 | 0 | 23 | 0.2 |
| OATMEAL W/ RAISINS COOKIES | 4 COOKIE | 10 | 245 | 36 | 3 | 2 | 52 | 2.5 |
| OATMEAL,CKD,INSTNT,FLVRD,FORTF | 1 PKT | 2 | 160 | 31 | 5 | 0 | 164 | 0.3 |
| OATMEAL,CKD,INSTNT,PLAIN,FORTF | 1 PKT | 2 | 105 | 18 | 4 | 0 | 177 | 0.3 |
| OATMEAL,CKD,RG,QCK,INST,W/OSAL | 1 CUP | 2 | 145 | 25 | 6 | 0 | 234 | 0.4 |
| OATMEAL,CKD,RG,QCK,INST,W/SALT | 1 CUP | 2 | 145 | 25 | 6 | 0 | 234 | 0.4 |
| OCEAN PERCH, BREADED, FRIED | 1 FILLET | 11 | 185 | 7 | 16 | 66 | 85 | 2.6 |
| OKRA PODS, COOKED | 8 PODS | 0 | 25 | 6 | 2 | 0 | 85 | 0 |
| OLIVE OIL | 1 CUP | 216 | 1910 | 0 | 0 | 0 | 216 | 29.2 |
| OLIVE OIL | 1 TBSP | 14 | 125 | 0 | 0 | 0 | 14 | 1.9 |
| OLIVES, CANNED, GREEN | 4 MEDIUM | 2 | 15 | 0 | 0 | 0 | 13 | 0.2 |
| OLIVES, CANNED, RIPE, MISSION | 3 SMALL | 2 | 15 | 0 | 0 | 0 | 9 | 0.3 |
| ONION POWDER | 1 TSP | 0 | 5 | 2 | 0 | 0 | 2.1 | 0 |
| ONION RINGS, BREADED,FRZN,PRPD | 2 RINGS | 5 | 80 | 8 | 1 | 0 | 20 | 1.7 |
| ONION SOUP, DEHYDRATD, PREPRED | 1 PKT | 0 | 20 | 4 | 1 | 0 | 184 | 0.1 |
| ONION SOUP, DEHYDRTD, UNPRPRED | 1 PKT | 0 | 20 | 4 | 1 | 0 | 7 | 0.1 |
| ONIONS, RAW, CHOPPED | 1 CUP | 0 | 55 | 12 | 2 | 0 | 160 | 0.1 |
| ONIONS, RAW, COOKED, DRAINED | 1 CUP | 0 | 60 | 13 | 2 | 0 | 210 | 0.1 |
| ONIONS, RAW, SLICED | 1 CUP | 0 | 40 | 8 | 1 | 0 | 115 | 0.1 |
| ONIONS, SPRING, RAW | 6 ONION | 0 | 10 | 2 | 1 | 0 | 30 | 0 |
| ORANGE JUICE, CANNED | 1 CUP | 0 | 105 | 25 | 1 | 0 | 249 | 0 |
| ORANGE JUICE, CHILLED | 1 CUP | 1 | 110 | 25 | 2 | 0 | 249 | 0.1 |
| ORANGE JUICE, RAW | 1 CUP | 0 | 110 | 26 | 2 | 0 | 248 | 0.1 |

| Description of food | Fat (Grams) | Food Energy (calories) | Carbohydrate (Grams) | Protein (Grams) | Cholesterol (Milligrams) | Weight (Grams) | Saturated Fat (Grams) |
|---|---|---|---|---|---|---|---|
| ORANGE JUICE,FROZEN CONCENTRTE6 FL OZ | 0 | 340 | 81 | 5 | 0 | 213 | 0.1 |
| ORANGE JUICE,FRZN,CNCN,DILUTED1 CUP | 0 | 110 | 27 | 2 | 0 | 249 | 0 |
| ORANGE SODA 12 FL OZ | 0 | 180 | 46 | 0 | 0 | 372 | 0 |
| ORANGE + GRAPEFRUIT JUCE,CANND1 CUP | 0 | 105 | 25 | 1 | 0 | 247 | 0 |
| ORANGES, RAW 1 ORANGE | 0 | 60 | 15 | 1 | 0 | 131 | 0 |
| ORANGES, RAW, SECTIONS 1 CUP | 0 | 85 | 21 | 2 | 0 | 180 | 0 |
| OREGANO 1 TSP | 0 | 5 | 1 | 0 | 0 | 1.5 | 0 |
| OYSTERS, BREADED, FRIED 1 OYSTER | 5 | 90 | 5 | 5 | 35 | 45 | 1.4 |
| OYSTERS, RAW 1 CUP | 4 | 160 | 8 | 20 | 120 | 240 | 1.4 |
| PANCAKES, BUCKWHEAT, FROM MIX 1 PANCAK | 2 | 55 | 6 | 2 | 20 | 27 | 0.9 |
| PANCAKES, PLAIN, FROM MIX 1 PANCAK | 2 | 60 | 8 | 2 | 16 | 27 | 0.5 |
| PANCAKES, PLAIN, HOME RECIPE 1 PANCAK | 2 | 60 | 9 | 2 | 16 | 27 | 0.5 |
| PAPAYAS, RAW 1 CUP | 0 | 65 | 17 | 1 | 0 | 140 | 0.1 |
| PAPRIKA 1 TSP | 0 | 5 | 1 | 0 | 0 | 2.1 | 0 |
| PARMESAN CHEESE, GRATED 1 CUP | 30 | 455 | 4 | 42 | 79 | 100 | 19.1 |
| PARMESAN CHEESE, GRATED 1 OZ | 9 | 130 | 1 | 12 | 22 | 28.35 | 5.4 |
| PARMESAN CHEESE, GRATED 1 TBSP | 2 | 25 | 0 | 2 | 4 | 5 | 1 |
| PARSLEY, FREEZE-DRIED 1 TBSP | 0 | 0 | 0 | 0 | 0 | 0.4 | 0 |
| PARSLEY, RAW 10 SPRIG | 0 | 5 | 1 | 0 | 0 | 10 | 0 |
| PARSNIPS, COOKED, DRAINED 1 CUP | 0 | 125 | 30 | 2 | 0 | 156 | 0.1 |
| PASTERZD PROCES CHEESE, SWISS 1 OZ | 7 | 95 | 1 | 7 | 24 | 28.35 | 4.5 |
| PASTERZD PROCES CHEESE,AMERICN1 OZ | 9 | 105 | 0 | 6 | 27 | 28.35 | 5.6 |
| PASTERZD PROCES CHESE FOOD,AMR1 OZ | 7 | 95 | 2 | 6 | 18 | 28.35 | 4.4 |
| PASTERZD PROCES CHESE SPRED,AM1 OZ | 6 | 80 | 2 | 5 | 16 | 28.35 | 3.8 |
| PEA BEANS, DRY, COOKED,DRAINED1 CUP | 1 | 225 | 40 | 15 | 0 | 190 | 0.1 |

120

| Description of food | | Fat (Grams) | Food Energy (calories) | Carbohydrate (Grams) | Protein (Grams) | Cholesterol (Milligrams) | Weight (Grams) | Saturated Fat (Grams) |
|---|---|---|---|---|---|---|---|---|
| PEACH PIE | 1 PIE | 101 | 2410 | 361 | 24 | 0 | 945 | 24.6 |
| PEACH PIE | 1 PIECE | 17 | 405 | 60 | 4 | 0 | 158 | 4.1 |
| PEACHES, CANNED, HEAVY SYRUP | 1 CUP | 0 | 190 | 51 | 1 | 0 | 256 | 0 |
| PEACHES, CANNED, HEAVY SYRUP | 1 HALF | 0 | 60 | 16 | 0 | 0 | 81 | 0 |
| PEACHES, CANNED, JUICE PACK | 1 CUP | 0 | 110 | 29 | 2 | 0 | 248 | 0 |
| PEACHES, CANNED, JUICE PACK | 1 HALF | 0 | 35 | 9 | 0 | 0 | 77 | 0 |
| PEACHES, DRIED | 1 CUP | 1 | 380 | 98 | 6 | 0 | 160 | 0.1 |
| PEACHES, DRIED,COOKED,UNSWETND | 1 CUP | 1 | 200 | 51 | 3 | 0 | 258 | 0.1 |
| PEACHES, FROZEN,SWETNED,W/VITC | 1 CUP | 0 | 235 | 60 | 2 | 0 | 250 | 0 |
| PEACHES, FROZEN,SWETNED,W/VITC | 10 OZ | 0 | 265 | 68 | 2 | 0 | 284 | 0 |
| PEACHES, RAW | 1 PEACH | 0 | 35 | 10 | 1 | 0 | 87 | 0 |
| PEACHES, RAW, SLICED | 1 CUP | 0 | 75 | 19 | 1 | 0 | 170 | 0 |
| PEANUT BUTTER | 1 TBSP | 8 | 95 | 3 | 5 | 0 | 16 | 1.4 |
| PEANUT BUTTER COOKIE,HOME RECP | 4 COOKIE | 14 | 245 | 28 | 4 | 22 | 48 | 4 |
| PEANUT OIL | 1 CUP | 216 | 1910 | 0 | 0 | 0 | 216 | 36.5 |
| PEANUT OIL | 1 TBSP | 14 | 125 | 0 | 0 | 0 | 14 | 2.4 |
| PEANUTS, OIL ROASTED, SALTED | 1 CUP | 71 | 840 | 27 | 39 | 0 | 145 | 9.9 |
| PEANUTS, OIL ROASTED, SALTED | 1 OZ | 14 | 165 | 5 | 8 | 0 | 28.35 | 1.9 |
| PEANUTS, OIL ROASTED, UNSALTED | 1 CUP | 71 | 840 | 27 | 39 | 0 | 145 | 9.9 |
| PEANUTS, OIL ROASTED, UNSALTED | 1 OZ | 14 | 165 | 5 | 8 | 0 | 28.35 | 1.9 |
| PEARS, CANNED, HEAVY SYRUP | 1 CUP | 0 | 190 | 49 | 1 | 0 | 255 | 0 |
| PEARS, CANNED, HEAVY SYRUP | 1 HALF | 0 | 60 | 15 | 0 | 0 | 79 | 0 |
| PEARS, CANNED, JUICE PACK | 1 CUP | 0 | 125 | 32 | 1 | 0 | 248 | 0 |
| PEARS, CANNED, JUICE PACK | 1 HALF | 0 | 40 | 10 | 0 | 0 | 77 | 0 |
| PEARS, RAW, BARTLETT | 1 PEAR | 1 | 100 | 25 | 1 | 0 | 166 | 0 |

| Description of food | | Fat (Grams) | Food Energy (calories) | Carbohydrate (Grams) | Protein (Grams) | Cholesterol (Milligrams) | Weight (Grams) | Saturated Fat (Grams) |
|---|---|---|---|---|---|---|---|---|
| PEARS, RAW, BOSC | 1 PEAR | 1 | 85 | 21 | 1 | 0 | 141 | 0 |
| PEARS, RAW, D'ANJOU | 1 PEAR | 1 | 120 | 30 | 1 | 0 | 200 | 0 |
| PEAS, EDIBLE POD, COOKED,DRNED | 1 CUP | 0 | 65 | 11 | 5 | 0 | 160 | 0.1 |
| PEAS, GREEN,CNND,DRND, W/ SALT | 1 CUP | 1 | 115 | 21 | 8 | 0 | 170 | 0.1 |
| PEAS, GREEN,CNND,DRND,W/O SALT | 1 CUP | 1 | 115 | 21 | 8 | 0 | 170 | 0.1 |
| PEAS, SPLIT, DRY, COOKED | 1 CUP | 1 | 230 | 42 | 16 | 0 | 200 | 0.1 |
| PEAS,GRN, FROZEN COOKED,DRANED | 1 CUP | 0 | 125 | 23 | 8 | 0 | 160 | 0.1 |
| PEA, GREEN, SOUP, CANNED | 1 CUP | 3 | 165 | 27 | 9 | 0 | 250 | 1.4 |
| PECAN PIE | 1 PIE | 189 | 3450 | 423 | 42 | 569 | 825 | 28.1 |
| PECAN PIE | 1 PIECE | 32 | 575 | 71 | 7 | 95 | 138 | 4.7 |
| PECANS, HALVES | 1 CUP | 73 | 720 | 20 | 8 | 0 | 108 | 5.9 |
| PECANS, HALVES | 1 OZ | 19 | 190 | 5 | 2 | 0 | 28.35 | 1.5 |
| PEPPER-TYPE SODA | 12 FL OZ | 0 | 160 | 41 | 0 | 0 | 369 | 0 |
| PEPPERS, HOT CHILI, RAW, GREEN | 1 PEPPER | 0 | 20 | 4 | 1 | 0 | 45 | 0 |
| PEPPERS, HOT CHILI, RAW, RED | 1 PEPPER | 0 | 20 | 4 | 1 | 0 | 45 | 0 |
| PEPPERS, SWEET, COOKED, GREEN | 1 PEPPER | 0 | 15 | 3 | 0 | 0 | 73 | 0 |
| PEPPERS, SWEET, COOKED, RED | 1 PEPPER | 0 | 15 | 3 | 0 | 0 | 73 | 0 |
| PEPPERS, SWEET, RAW, GREEN | 1 PEPPER | 0 | 20 | 4 | 1 | 0 | 74 | 0 |
| PEPPERS, SWEET, RAW, RED | 1 PEPPER | 0 | 20 | 4 | 1 | 0 | 74 | 0 |
| PEPPER, BLACK | 1 TSP | 0 | 5 | 1 | 0 | 0 | 2.1 | 0 |
| PICKLES, CUCUMBER, DILL | 1 PICKLE | 0 | 5 | 1 | 0 | 0 | 65 | 0 |
| PICKLES, CUCUMBER, FRESH PACK | 2 SLICES | 0 | 10 | 3 | 0 | 0 | 15 | 0 |
| PICKLES, CUCUMBER, SWT GHERKIN | 1 PICKLE | 0 | 20 | 5 | 0 | 0 | 15 | 0 |
| PIECRUST, FROM MIX | 2 CRUST | 93 | 1485 | 141 | 20 | 0 | 320 | 22.7 |
| PIECRUST,FROM HOME RECIPE | 1 SHELL | 60 | 900 | 79 | 11 | 0 | 180 | 14.8 |

| Description of food | | Fat (Grams) | Food Energy (calories) | Carbohydrate (Grams) | Protein (Grams) | Cholesterol (Milligrams) | Weight (Grams) | Saturated Fat (Grams) |
|---|---|---|---|---|---|---|---|---|
| PINE NUTS | 1 OZ | 17 | 160 | 5 | 3 | 0 | 28.35 | 2.7 |
| PINEAPPLE-GRAPEFRUIT JUICEDRNK | 6 FL OZ | 0 | 90 | 23 | 0 | 0 | 187 | 0 |
| PINEAPPLE JUICE, CANNED, UNSWTN | 1 CUP | 0 | 140 | 34 | 1 | 0 | 250 | 0 |
| PINEAPPLE, CANNED, HEAVY SYRUP | 1 CUP | 0 | 200 | 52 | 1 | 0 | 255 | 0 |
| PINEAPPLE, CANNED, HEAVY SYRUP | 1 SLICE | 0 | 45 | 12 | 0 | 0 | 58 | 0 |
| PINEAPPLE, CANNED, JUICE PACK | 1 CUP | 0 | 150 | 39 | 1 | 0 | 250 | 0 |
| PINEAPPLE, CANNED, JUICE PACK | 1 SLICE | 0 | 35 | 9 | 0 | 0 | 58 | 0 |
| PINEAPPLE, RAW, DICED | 1 CUP | 1 | 75 | 19 | 1 | 0 | 155 | 0 |
| PINTO BEANS,DRY,COOKED,DRAINED | 1 CUP | 1 | 265 | 49 | 15 | 0 | 180 | 0.1 |
| PISTACHIO NUTS | 1 OZ | 14 | 165 | 7 | 6 | 0 | 28.35 | 1.7 |
| PITA BREAD | 1 PITA | 1 | 165 | 33 | 6 | 0 | 60 | 0.1 |
| PIZZA, CHEESE | 1 SLICE | 9 | 290 | 39 | 15 | 56 | 120 | 4.1 |
| PLANTAINS, COOKED | 1 CUP | 0 | 180 | 48 | 1 | 0 | 154 | 0.1 |
| PLANTAINS, RAW | 1 PLANTN | 1 | 220 | 57 | 2 | 0 | 179 | 0.3 |
| PLUMS, CANNED, HEAVY SYRUP | 1 CUP | 0 | 230 | 60 | 1 | 0 | 258 | 0 |
| PLUMS, CANNED, HEAVY SYRUP | 3 PLUMS | 0 | 120 | 31 | 0 | 0 | 133 | 0 |
| PLUMS, CANNED, JUICE PACK | 1 CUP | 0 | 145 | 38 | 1 | 0 | 252 | 0 |
| PLUMS, CANNED, JUICE PACK | 3 PLUMS | 0 | 55 | 14 | 0 | 0 | 95 | 0 |
| PLUMS, RAW, 1-1/2-IN DIAM | 1 PLUM | 0 | 15 | 4 | 0 | 0 | 28 | 0 |
| PLUMS, RAW, 2-1/8-IN DIAM | 1 PLUM | 0 | 35 | 9 | 1 | 0 | 66 | 0 |
| POPCORN, AIR-POPPED, UNSALTED | 1 CUP | 0 | 30 | 6 | 1 | 0 | 8 | 0 |
| POPCORN, POPPED, VEG OIL,SALTD | 1 CUP | 3 | 55 | 6 | 1 | 0 | 11 | 0.5 |
| POPCORN, SUGAR SYRUP COATED | 1 CUP | 1 | 135 | 30 | 2 | 0 | 35 | 0.1 |
| POPSICLE | 1 POPCLE | 0 | 70 | 18 | 0 | 0 | 95 | 0 |
| PORK CHOP, LOIN, BROIL, LEAN | 2.5 OZ | 8 | 165 | 0 | 23 | 71 | 72 | 2.6 |

| Description of food | Fat (Grams) | Food Energy (calories) | Carbohydrate (Grams) | Protein (Grams) | Cholesterol (Milligrams) | Weight (Grams) | Saturated Fat (Grams) |
|---|---|---|---|---|---|---|---|
| PORK CHOP, LOIN, BROIL, LEN+FT3.1 OZ | 19 | 275 | 0 | 24 | 84 | 87 | 7 |
| PORK CHOP, LOIN,PANFRY, LEAN 2.4 OZ | 11 | 180 | 0 | 19 | 72 | 67 | 3.7 |
| PORK CHOP, LOIN,PANFRY,LEAN+FT3.1 OZ | 27 | 335 | 0 | 21 | 92 | 89 | 9.8 |
| PORK FRESH HAM, ROASTD, LEAN 2.5 OZ | 8 | 160 | 0 | 20 | 68 | 72 | 2.7 |
| PORK FRESH HAM, ROASTD,LEAN+FT3 OZ | 18 | 250 | 0 | 21 | 79 | 85 | 6.4 |
| PORK FRESH RIB, ROASTD, LEAN 2.5 OZ | 10 | 175 | 0 | 20 | 56 | 71 | 3.4 |
| PORK FRESH RIB, ROASTD,LEAN+FT3 OZ | 20 | 270 | 0 | 21 | 69 | 85 | 7.2 |
| PORK SHOULDER, BRAISD, LEAN 2.4 OZ | 8 | 165 | 0 | 22 | 76 | 67 | 2.8 |
| PORK SHOULDER, BRAISD,LEAN+FAT3 OZ | 22 | 295 | 0 | 23 | 93 | 85 | 7.9 |
| PORK, CURED, BACON, REGUL,CKED3 SLICE | 9 | 110 | 0 | 6 | 16 | 19 | 3.3 |
| PORK, CURED, BACON,CANADN,CKED2 SLICE | 4 | 85 | 1 | 11 | 27 | 46 | 1.3 |
| PORK, CURED, HAM, CANNED,ROAST3 OZ | 7 | 140 | 0 | 18 | 35 | 85 | 2.4 |
| PORK, CURED, HAM, ROSTED,LEAN 2.4 OZ | 4 | 105 | 0 | 17 | 37 | 68 | 1.3 |
| PORK, CURED, HAM, ROSTED,LN+FT3 OZ | 14 | 205 | 0 | 18 | 53 | 85 | 5.1 |
| PORK, LINK, COOKED 1 LINK | 4 | 50 | 0 | 3 | 11 | 13 | 1.4 |
| PORK, LUNCHEON MEAT,CANNED 2 SLICES | 13 | 140 | 1 | 5 | 26 | 42 | 4.5 |
| PORK, LUNCHEON MEAT,CHOPPD HAM2 SLICES | 7 | 95 | 0 | 7 | 21 | 42 | 2.4 |
| PORK, LUNCHEON MEAT,CKD HAM,LN2 SLICES | 3 | 75 | 1 | 11 | 27 | 57 | 0.9 |
| PORK, LUNCHEON MEAT,CKD HAM,RG2 SLICES | 6 | 105 | 2 | 10 | 32 | 57 | 1.9 |
| POTATO CHIPS 10 CHIPS | 7 | 105 | 10 | 1 | 0 | 20 | 1.8 |
| POTATO SALAD MADE W/ MAYONNAIS1 CUP | 21 | 360 | 28 | 7 | 170 | 250 | 3.6 |
| POTATOES, AU GRATIN, FROM MIX 1 CUP | 10 | 230 | 31 | 6 | 12 | 245 | 6.3 |
| POTATOES, AU GRATIN, HOME RECP1 CUP | 19 | 325 | 28 | 12 | 56 | 245 | 11.6 |
| POTATOES, BAKED FLESH ONLY 1 POTATO | 0 | 145 | 34 | 3 | 0 | 156 | 0 |
| POTATOES, BAKED WITH SKIN 1 POTATO | 0 | 220 | 51 | 5 | 0 | 202 | 0.1 |

| Description of food | Fat (Grams) | Food Energy (calories) | Carbohydrate (Grams) | Protein (Grams) | Cholesterol (Milligrams) | Weight (Grams) | Saturated Fat (Grams) |
|---|---|---|---|---|---|---|---|
| POTATOES, BOILED, PEELED AFTER 1 POTATO | 0 | 120 | 27 | 3 | 0 | 136 | 0 |
| POTATOES, BOILED, PEELED BEFOR 1 POTATO | 0 | 115 | 27 | 2 | 0 | 135 | 0 |
| POTATOES, HASHED BROWN,FR FRZN 1 CUP | 18 | 340 | 44 | 5 | 0 | 156 | 7 |
| POTATOES, MASHED,FRM DEHYDRTED 1 CUP | 12 | 235 | 32 | 4 | 29 | 210 | 7.2 |
| POTATOES, MASHED,RECPE,MLK+MAR 1 CUP | 9 | 225 | 35 | 4 | 4 | 210 | 2.2 |
| POTATOES, MASHED,RECPE,W/ MILK 1 CUP | 1 | 160 | 37 | 4 | 4 | 210 | 0.7 |
| POTATOES, SCALLOPED, FROM MIX 1 CUP | 11 | 230 | 31 | 5 | 27 | 245 | 6.5 |
| POTATOES, SCALLOPED, HOME RECP 1 CUP | 9 | 210 | 26 | 7 | 29 | 245 | 5.5 |
| POTATOES,FRENCH-FRD,FRZN,FRIED 10 STRIP | 8 | 160 | 20 | 2 | 0 | 50 | 2.5 |
| POTATOES,FRENCH-FRD,FRZN,OVEN 10 STRIP | 4 | 110 | 17 | 2 | 0 | 50 | 2.1 |
| POUND CAKE, COMMERCIAL 1 LOAF | 94 | 1935 | 257 | 26 | 1100 | 500 | 52 |
| POUND CAKE, COMMERCIAL 1 SLICE | 5 | 110 | 15 | 2 | 64 | 29 | 3 |
| POUND CAKE, FROM HOME RECIPE 1 LOAF | 94 | 2025 | 265 | 33 | 555 | 514 | 21.1 |
| POUND CAKE, FROM HOME RECIPE 1 SLICE | 5 | 120 | 15 | 2 | 32 | 30 | 1.2 |
| PRETZELS, STICK 10 PRETZ | 0 | 10 | 2 | 0 | 0 | 3 | 0 |
| PRETZELS, TWISTED, DUTCH 1 PRETZ | 1 | 65 | 13 | 2 | 0 | 16 | 0.1 |
| PRETZELS, TWISTED, THIN 10 PRETZ | 2 | 240 | 48 | 6 | 0 | 60 | 0.4 |
| PRODUCT 19 CEREAL 1 OZ | 0 | 110 | 24 | 3 | 0 | 28.35 | 0 |
| PROVOLONE CHEESE 1 OZ | 8 | 100 | 1 | 7 | 20 | 28.35 | 4.8 |
| PRUNE JUICE, CANNED 1 CUP | 0 | 180 | 45 | 2 | 0 | 256 | 0 |
| PRUNES, DRIED 5 LARGE | 0 | 115 | 31 | 1 | 0 | 49 | 0 |
| PRUNES, DRIED, COOKED,UNSWTNED 1 CUP | 0 | 225 | 60 | 2 | 0 | 212 | 0 |
| PUDDING, CHOCOLATE,CANNED 5 OZ | 11 | 205 | 30 | 3 | 1 | 142 | 9.5 |
| PUDDING, CHOC, COOKED FROM MIX 1/2 CUP | 4 | 150 | 25 | 4 | 15 | 130 | 2.4 |
| PUDDING, CHOC, INSTANT, FR MIX 1/2 CUP | 4 | 155 | 27 | 4 | 14 | 130 | 2.3 |

| Description of food | | Fat (Grams) | Food Energy (calories) | Carbohydrate (Grams) | Protein (Grams) | Cholesterol (Milligrams) | Weight (Grams) | Saturated Fat (Grams) |
|---|---|---|---|---|---|---|---|---|
| PUDDING, RICE, FROM MIX | 1/2 CUP | 4 | 155 | 27 | 4 | 15 | 132 | 2.3 |
| PUDDING, TAPIOCA, CANNED | 5 OZ | 5 | 160 | 28 | 3 | 0 | 142 | 4.8 |
| PUDDING, TAPIOCA, FROM MIX | 1/2 CUP | 4 | 145 | 25 | 4 | 15 | 130 | 2.3 |
| PUDDING, VANILLA, CANNED | 5 OZ | 10 | 220 | 33 | 2 | 1 | 142 | 9.5 |
| PUDDING, VNLLA,COOKED FROM MIX | 1/2 CUP | 4 | 145 | 25 | 4 | 15 | 130 | 2.3 |
| PUDDING, VNLLA,INSTANT FRM MIX | 1/2 CUP | 4 | 150 | 27 | 4 | 15 | 130 | 2.2 |
| PUMPERNICKEL BREAD | 1 LOAF | 16 | 1160 | 218 | 42 | 0 | 454 | 2.6 |
| PUMPERNICKEL BREAD | 1 SLICE | 1 | 80 | 16 | 3 | 0 | 32 | 0.2 |
| PUMPERNICKEL BREAD, TOASTED | 1 SLICE | 1 | 80 | 16 | 3 | 0 | 29 | 0.2 |
| PUMPKIN AND SQUASH KERNELS | 1 OZ | 13 | 155 | 5 | 7 | 0 | 28.35 | 2.5 |
| PUMPKIN PIE | 1 PIE | 102 | 1920 | 223 | 36 | 655 | 910 | 38.2 |
| PUMPKIN PIE | 1 PIECE | 17 | 320 | 37 | 6 | 109 | 152 | 6.4 |
| PUMPKIN, CANNED | 1 CUP | 1 | 85 | 20 | 3 | 0 | 245 | 0.4 |
| PUMPKIN, COOKED FROM RAW | 1 CUP | 0 | 50 | 12 | 2 | 0 | 245 | 0.1 |
| QUICHE LORRAINE | 1 SLICE | 48 | 600 | 29 | 13 | 285 | 176 | 23.2 |
| RADISHES, RAW | 4 RADISH | 0 | 5 | 1 | 0 | 0 | 18 | 0 |
| RAISIN BRAN, KELLOGG'S | 1 OZ | 1 | 90 | 21 | 3 | 0 | 28.35 | 0.1 |
| RAISIN BRAN, POST | 1 OZ | 1 | 85 | 21 | 3 | 0 | 28.35 | 0.1 |
| RAISIN BREAD | 1 LOAF | 18 | 1260 | 239 | 37 | 0 | 454 | 4.1 |
| RAISIN BREAD | 1 SLICE | 1 | 65 | 13 | 2 | 0 | 25 | 0.2 |
| RAISIN BREAD, TOASTED | 1 SLICE | 1 | 65 | 13 | 2 | 0 | 21 | 0.2 |
| RAISINS | 1 CUP | 1 | 435 | 115 | 5 | 0 | 145 | 0.2 |
| RAISINS | 1 PACKET | 0 | 40 | 11 | 0 | 0 | 14 | 0 |
| RASPBERRIES, FROZEN, SWEETENED | 1 CUP | 0 | 255 | 65 | 2 | 0 | 250 | 0 |
| RASPBERRIES, FROZEN, SWEETENED | 10 OZ | 0 | 295 | 74 | 2 | 0 | 284 | 0 |

| Description of food | | Fat (Grams) | Food Energy (calories) | Carbohydrate (Grams) | Protein (Grams) | Cholesterol (Milligrams) | Weight (Grams) | Saturated Fat (Grams) |
|---|---|---|---|---|---|---|---|---|
| RASPBERRIES, RAW | 1 CUP | 1 | 60 | 14 | 1 | 0 | 123 | 0 |
| RED KIDNEY BEANS, DRY, CANNED | 1 CUP | 1 | 230 | 42 | 15 | 0 | 255 | 0.1 |
| REFRIED BEANS, CANNED | 1 CUP | 3 | 295 | 51 | 18 | 0 | 290 | 0.4 |
| RELISH, SWEET | 1 TBSP | 0 | 20 | 5 | 0 | 0 | 15 | 0 |
| RHUBARB, COOKED, ADDED SUGAR | 1 CUP | 0 | 280 | 75 | 1 | 0 | 240 | 0 |
| RICE KRISPIES CEREAL | 1 OZ | 0 | 110 | 25 | 2 | 0 | 28.35 | 0 |
| RICE, BROWN, COOKED | 1 CUP | 1 | 230 | 50 | 5 | 0 | 195 | 0.3 |
| RICE, WHITE, COOKED | 1 CUP | 0 | 225 | 50 | 4 | 0 | 205 | 0.1 |
| RICE, WHITE, INSTANT, COOKED | 1 CUP | 0 | 180 | 40 | 4 | 0 | 165 | 0.1 |
| RICE, WHITE, PARBOILED, COOKED | 1 CUP | 0 | 185 | 41 | 4 | 0 | 175 | 0 |
| RICE, WHITE, PARBOILED, RAW | 1 CUP | 1 | 685 | 150 | 14 | 0 | 185 | 0.1 |
| RICE, WHITE, RAW | 1 CUP | 1 | 670 | 149 | 12 | 0 | 185 | 0.2 |
| RICOTTA CHEESE, PART SKIM MILK | 1 CUP | 19 | 340 | 13 | 28 | 76 | 246 | 12.1 |
| RICOTTA CHEESE, WHOLE MILK | 1 CUP | 32 | 430 | 7 | 28 | 124 | 246 | 20.4 |
| ROAST BEEF SANDWICH | 1 SANDWH | 13 | 345 | 34 | 22 | 55 | 150 | 3.5 |
| ROLLS, DINNER, COMMERCIAL | 1 ROLL | 2 | 85 | 14 | 2 | 0 | 28 | 0.5 |
| ROLLS, DINNER, HOME RECIPE | 1 ROLL | 3 | 120 | 20 | 3 | 12 | 35 | 0.8 |
| ROLLS, FRANKFURTER + HAMBURGER | 1 ROLL | 2 | 115 | 20 | 3 | 0 | 40 | 0.5 |
| ROLLS, HARD | 1 ROLL | 2 | 155 | 30 | 5 | 0 | 50 | 0.4 |
| ROLLS, HOAGIE OR SUBMARINE | 1 ROLL | 8 | 400 | 72 | 11 | 0 | 135 | 1.8 |
| ROOT BEER | 12 FL OZ | 0 | 165 | 42 | 0 | 0 | 370 | 0 |
| RYE BREAD, LIGHT | 1 LOAF | 17 | 1190 | 218 | 38 | 0 | 454 | 3.3 |
| RYE BREAD, LIGHT | 1 SLICE | 1 | 65 | 12 | 2 | 0 | 25 | 0.2 |
| RYE BREAD, LIGHT, TOASTED | 1 SLICE | 1 | 65 | 12 | 2 | 0 | 22 | 0.2 |
| RYE WAFERS, WHOLE-GRAIN | 2 WAFERS | 1 | 55 | 10 | 1 | 0 | 14 | 0.3 |

| Description of food | | Fat (Grams) | Food Energy (calories) | Carbohydrate (Grams) | Protein (Grams) | Cholesterol (Milligrams) | Weight (Grams) | Saturated Fat (Grams) |
|---|---|---|---|---|---|---|---|---|
| SAFFLOWER OIL | 1 CUP | 218 | 1925 | 0 | 0 | 0 | 218 | 19.8 |
| SAFFLOWER OIL | 1 TBSP | 14 | 125 | 0 | 0 | 0 | 14 | 1.3 |
| SALAMI, COOKED TYPE | 2 SLICES | 11 | 145 | 1 | 8 | 37 | 57 | 4.6 |
| SALAMI, DRY TYPE | 2 SLICES | 7 | 85 | 1 | 5 | 16 | 20 | 2.4 |
| SALMON, BAKED, RED | 3 OZ | 5 | 140 | 0 | 21 | 60 | 85 | 1.2 |
| SALMON, CANNED, PINK, W/ BONES | 3 OZ | 5 | 120 | 0 | 17 | 34 | 85 | 0.9 |
| SALMON, SMOKED | 3 OZ | 8 | 150 | 0 | 18 | 51 | 85 | 2.6 |
| SALT | 1 TSP | 0 | 0 | 0 | 0 | 0 | 5.5 | 0 |
| SALTINES | 4 CRACKR | 1 | 50 | 9 | 1 | 4 | 12 | 0.5 |
| SANDWICH SPREAD, PORK, BEEF | 1 TBSP | 3 | 35 | 2 | 1 | 6 | 15 | 0.9 |
| SANDWICH TYPE COOKIE | 4 COOKIE | 8 | 195 | 29 | 2 | 0 | 40 | 2 |
| SARDINES, ATLNTC,CNNED,OIL,DRN | 3 OZ | 9 | 175 | 0 | 20 | 85 | 85 | 2.1 |
| SAUERKRAUT, CANNED | 1 CUP | 0 | 45 | 10 | 2 | 0 | 236 | 0.1 |
| SCALLOPS, BREADED, FRZN,REHEAT | 6 SCALOP | 10 | 195 | 10 | 15 | 70 | 90 | 2.5 |
| SEAWEED, KELP, RAW | 1 OZ | 0 | 10 | 3 | 0 | 0 | 28.35 | 0.1 |
| SEAWEED, SPIRULINA, DRIED | 1 OZ | 2 | 80 | 7 | 16 | 0 | 28.35 | 0.8 |
| SELF-RISING FLOUR, UNSIFTED | 1 CUP | 1 | 440 | 93 | 12 | 0 | 125 | 0.2 |
| SEMISWEET CHOCOLATE | 1 CUP | 61 | 860 | 97 | 7 | 0 | 170 | 36.2 |
| SESAME SEEDS | 1 TBSP | 4 | 45 | 1 | 2 | 0 | 8 | 0.6 |
| SHAKES, THICK, CHOCOLATE | 10 OZ | 8 | 335 | 60 | 9 | 30 | 283 | 4.8 |
| SHAKES, THICK, VANILLA | 10 OZ | 9 | 315 | 50 | 11 | 33 | 283 | 5.3 |
| SHEETCAKE W/O FRSTNG,HOMERECIP | 1 CAKE | 108 | 2830 | 434 | 35 | 552 | 777 | 29.5 |
| SHEETCAKE,W/ WHFRSTNG,HOMERCIP | 1 CAKE | 129 | 4020 | 694 | 37 | 636 | 1096 | 41.6 |
| SHEETCAKE,W/ WHFRSTNG,HOMERECIP | 1 PIECE | 14 | 445 | 77 | 4 | 70 | 121 | 4.6 |
| SHEETCAKE,W/O FRSTNG,HOMERECIP | 1 PIECE | 12 | 315 | 48 | 4 | 61 | 86 | 3.3 |

| Description of food | | Fat (Grams) | Food Energy (calories) | Carbohydrate (Grams) | Protein (Grams) | Cholesterol (Milligrams) | Weight (Grams) | Saturated Fat (Grams) |
|---|---|---|---|---|---|---|---|---|
| SHERBET, 2% FAT | 1 CUP | 4 | 270 | 59 | 2 | 14 | 193 | 2.4 |
| SHERBET, 2% FAT | 1/2 GAL | 31 | 2160 | 469 | 17 | 113 | 1542 | 19 |
| SHORTBREAD COOKIE, COMMERCIAL 4 COOKIE | | 8 | 155 | 20 | 2 | 27 | 32 | 2.9 |
| SHORTBREAD COOKIE, HOME RECIPE2 COOKIE | | 8 | 145 | 17 | 2 | 0 | 28 | 1.3 |
| SHREDDED WHEAT CEREAL | 1 OZ | 1 | 100 | 23 | 3 | 0 | 28.35 | 0.1 |
| SHRIMP, CANNED, DRAINED | 3 OZ | 1 | 100 | 1 | 21 | 128 | 85 | 0.2 |
| SHRIMP, FRENCH FRIED | 3 OZ | 10 | 200 | 11 | 16 | 168 | 85 | 2.5 |
| SNACK CAKES,DEVILS FOOD,CREMFLSM CAKE | | 4 | 105 | 17 | 1 | 15 | 28 | 1.7 |
| SNACK CAKES,SPONGE CREME FLLNGSM CAKE | | 5 | 155 | 27 | 1 | 7 | 42 | 2.3 |
| SNACK TYPE CRACKERS | 1 CRACKR | 1 | 15 | 2 | 0 | 0 | 3 | 0.2 |
| SNAP BEAN,CNND,DRND,GREEN,SALT1 CUP | | 0 | 25 | 6 | 2 | 0 | 135 | 0 |
| SNAP BEAN,CNND,DRND,GRN,NOSALT1 CUP | | 0 | 25 | 6 | 2 | 0 | 135 | 0 |
| SNAP BEAN,CNND,DRND,YLLW, SALT1 CUP | | 0 | 25 | 6 | 2 | 0 | 135 | 0 |
| SNAP BEAN,CNND,DRND,YLLW,NOSAL1 CUP | | 0 | 25 | 6 | 2 | 0 | 135 | 0 |
| SNAP BEAN,FRZ,CKD,DRND,GREEN | 1 CUP | 0 | 35 | 8 | 2 | 0 | 135 | 0 |
| SNAP BEAN,FRZ,CKD,DRND,YELLOW | 1 CUP | 0 | 35 | 8 | 2 | 0 | 135 | 0 |
| SNAP BEAN,RAW,CKD,DRND,GREEN | 1 CUP | 0 | 45 | 10 | 2 | 0 | 125 | 0.1 |
| SNAP BEAN,RAW,CKD,DRND,YELLOW | 1 CUP | 0 | 45 | 10 | 2 | 0 | 125 | 0.1 |
| SOUR CREAM | 1 CUP | 48 | 495 | 10 | 7 | 102 | 230 | 30 |
| SOUR CREAM | 1 TBSP | 3 | 25 | 1 | 0 | 5 | 12 | 1.6 |
| SOY SAUCE | 1 TBSP | 0 | 10 | 2 | 2 | 0 | 18 | 0 |
| SOYBEAN-COTTONSEED OIL, HYDRGN1 CUP | | 218 | 1925 | 0 | 0 | 0 | 218 | 39.2 |
| SOYBEAN-COTTONSEED OIL, HYDRGN1 TBSP | | 14 | 125 | 0 | 0 | 0 | 14 | 2.5 |
| SOYBEAN OIL, HYDROGENATED | 1 CUP | 218 | 1925 | 0 | 0 | 0 | 218 | 32.5 |
| SOYBEAN OIL, HYDROGENATED | 1 TBSP | 14 | 125 | 0 | 0 | 0 | 14 | 2.1 |

| Description of food | Fat (Grams) | Food Energy (calories) | Carbohydrate (Grams) | Protein (Grams) | Cholesterol (Milligrams) | Weight (Grams) | Saturated Fat (Grams) |
|---|---|---|---|---|---|---|---|
| SOYBEANS, DRY, COOKED, DRAINED 1 CUP | 10 | 235 | 19 | 20 | 0 | 180 | 1.3 |
| SPAGHETTI, COOKED, FIRM 1 CUP | 1 | 190 | 39 | 7 | 0 | 130 | 0.1 |
| SPAGHETTI, COOKED, TENDER 1 CUP | 1 | 155 | 32 | 5 | 0 | 140 | 0.1 |
| SPAGHETTI, TOM SAUCE CHEES,CND 1 CUP | 2 | 190 | 39 | 6 | 3 | 250 | 0.4 |
| SPAGHETTI, TOM SAUCE CHEE, HMRP 1 CUP | 9 | 260 | 37 | 9 | 8 | 250 | 3 |
| SPAGHETTI,MEATBALLS,TOMSAC,CND 1 CUP | 10 | 260 | 29 | 12 | 23 | 250 | 2.4 |
| SPAGHETTI,MEATBALLS,TOMSA,HMRP 1 CUP | 12 | 330 | 39 | 19 | 89 | 248 | 3.9 |
| SPECIAL K CEREAL 1 OZ | 0 | 110 | 21 | 6 | 0 | 28.35 | 0 |
| SPINACH SOUFFLE 1 CUP | 18 | 220 | 3 | 11 | 184 | 136 | 7.1 |
| SPINACH, CANNED, DRND,W/ SALT 1 CUP | 1 | 50 | 7 | 6 | 0 | 214 | 0.2 |
| SPINACH, CANNED, DRND,W/O SALT 1 CUP | 1 | 50 | 7 | 6 | 0 | 214 | 0.2 |
| SPINACH, COOKED FR FRZEN, DRND 1 CUP | 0 | 55 | 10 | 6 | 0 | 190 | 0.1 |
| SPINACH, COOKED FROM RAW, DRND 1 CUP | 0 | 40 | 7 | 5 | 0 | 180 | 0.1 |
| SPINACH, RAW 1 CUP | 0 | 10 | 2 | 2 | 0 | 55 | 0 |
| SQUASH, SUMMER, COOKED, DRAIND 1 CUP | 1 | 35 | 8 | 2 | 0 | 180 | 0.1 |
| SQUASH, WINTER, BAKED 1 CUP | 1 | 80 | 18 | 2 | 0 | 205 | 0.3 |
| STRAWBERRIES, FROZEN, SWEETEND 1 CUP | 0 | 245 | 66 | 1 | 0 | 255 | 0 |
| STRAWBERRIES, FROZEN, SWEETEND 10 OZ | 0 | 275 | 74 | 2 | 0 | 284 | 0 |
| STRAWBERRIES, RAW 1 CUP | 1 | 45 | 10 | 1 | 0 | 149 | 0 |
| SUGAR COOKIE, FROM REFRIG DOGH 4 COOKIE | 12 | 235 | 31 | 2 | 29 | 48 | 2.3 |
| SUGAR FROSTED FLAKES, KELLOGG 1 OZ | 0 | 110 | 26 | 1 | 0 | 28.35 | 0 |
| SUGAR SMACKS CEREAL 1 OZ | 1 | 105 | 25 | 2 | 0 | 28.35 | 0.1 |
| SUGAR, BROWN, PRESSED DOWN 1 CUP | 0 | 820 | 212 | 0 | 0 | 220 | 0 |
| SUGAR, POWDERED, SIFTED 1 CUP | 0 | 385 | 100 | 0 | 0 | 100 | 0 |
| SUGAR, WHITE, GRANULATED 1 CUP | 0 | 770 | 199 | 0 | 0 | 200 | 0 |

| Description of food | | Fat (Grams) | Food Energy (calories) | Carbohydrate (Grams) | Protein (Grams) | Cholesterol (Milligrams) | Weight (Grams) | Saturated Fat (Grams) |
|---|---|---|---|---|---|---|---|---|
| SUGAR, WHITE, GRANULATED | 1 PKT | 0 | 25 | 6 | 0 | 0 | 6 | 0 |
| SUGAR, WHITE, GRANULATED | 1 TBSP | 0 | 45 | 12 | 0 | 0 | 12 | 0 |
| SUNFLOWER OIL | 1 CUP | 218 | 1925 | 0 | 0 | 0 | 218 | 22.5 |
| SUNFLOWER OIL | 1 TBSP | 14 | 125 | 0 | 0 | 0 | 14 | 1.4 |
| SUNFLOWER SEEDS | 1 OZ | 14 | 160 | 5 | 6 | 0 | 28.35 | 1.5 |
| SUPER SUGAR CRISP CEREAL | 1 OZ | 0 | 105 | 26 | 2 | 0 | 28.35 | 0 |
| SWEET (DARK) CHOCOLATE | 1 OZ | 10 | 150 | 16 | 1 | 0 | 28.35 | 5.9 |
| SWEETENED CONDENSED MILK CNND | 1 CUP | 27 | 980 | 166 | 24 | 104 | 306 | 16.8 |
| SWEETPOTATOES, BAKED, PEELED | 1 POTATO | 0 | 115 | 28 | 2 | 0 | 114 | 0 |
| SWEETPOTATOES, BOILED W/O PEEL | 1 POTATO | 0 | 160 | 37 | 2 | 0 | 151 | 0.1 |
| SWEETPOTATOES, CANDIED | 1 PIECE | 3 | 145 | 29 | 1 | 8 | 105 | 1.4 |
| SWEETPOTATOES, CANNED, MASHED | 1 CUP | 1 | 260 | 59 | 5 | 0 | 255 | 0.1 |
| SWEETPOTATOES, CNNED, VAC PACK | 1 PIECE | 0 | 35 | 8 | 1 | 0 | 40 | 0 |
| SWISS CHEESE | 1 OZ | 8 | 105 | 1 | 8 | 26 | 28.35 | 5 |
| SYRUP, CHOCOLATE FLAVORED THIN | 2 TBSP | 0 | 85 | 22 | 1 | 0 | 38 | 0.2 |
| SYRUP, CHOCOLATE FLVRED, FUDGE | 2 TBSP | 5 | 125 | 21 | 2 | 0 | 38 | 3.1 |
| TABLE SYRUP (CORN AND MAPLE) | 2 TBSP | 0 | 122 | 32 | 0 | 0 | 42 | 0 |
| TACO | 1 TACO | 11 | 195 | 15 | 9 | 21 | 81 | 4.1 |
| TAHINI | 1 TBSP | 8 | 90 | 3 | 3 | 0 | 15 | 1.1 |
| TANGERINE JUICE, CANNED,SWTNED | 1 CUP | 0 | 125 | 30 | 1 | 0 | 249 | 0 |
| TANGERINES, CANNED, LIGHT SYRP | 1 CUP | 0 | 155 | 41 | 1 | 0 | 252 | 0 |
| TANGERINES, RAW | 1 TANGRN | 0 | 35 | 9 | 1 | 0 | 84 | 0 |
| TARTAR SAUCE | 1 TBSP | 8 | 75 | 1 | 0 | 4 | 14 | 1.2 |
| TEA, BREWED | 8 FL OZ | 0 | 0 | 0 | 0 | 0 | 240 | 0 |
| TEA, INSTANT,PREPRD,UNSWEETEND | 8 FL OZ | 0 | 0 | 1 | 0 | 0 | 241 | 0 |

| Description of food | Fat (Grams) | Food Energy (calories) | Carbohydrate (Grams) | Protein (Grams) | Cholesterol (Milligrams) | Weight (Grams) | Saturated Fat (Grams) |
|---|---|---|---|---|---|---|---|
| TEA,INSTANT,PREPARD,SWEETENED 8 FL OZ | 0 | 85 | 22 | 0 | 0 | 262 | 0 |
| TOASTER PASTRIES 1 PASTRY | 6 | 210 | 38 | 2 | 0 | 54 | 1.7 |
| TOFU 1 PIECE | 5 | 85 | 3 | 9 | 0 | 120 | 0.7 |
| TOMATO JUICE, CANNED WITH SALT 1 CUP | 0 | 40 | 10 | 2 | 0 | 244 | 0 |
| TOMATO JUICE, CANNED W/O SALT 1 CUP | 0 | 40 | 10 | 2 | 0 | 244 | 0 |
| TOMATO PASTE, CANNED WITH SALT 1 CUP | 2 | 220 | 49 | 10 | 0 | 262 | 0.3 |
| TOMATO PASTE, CANNED W/O SALT 1 CUP | 2 | 220 | 49 | 10 | 0 | 262 | 0.3 |
| TOMATO PUREE, CANNED WITH SALT 1 CUP | 0 | 105 | 25 | 4 | 0 | 250 | 0 |
| TOMATO PUREE, CANNED W/O SALT 1 CUP | 0 | 105 | 25 | 4 | 0 | 250 | 0 |
| TOMATO SAUCE, CANNED WITH SALT 1 CUP | 0 | 75 | 18 | 3 | 0 | 245 | 0.1 |
| TOMATO SOUP WITH MILK, CANNED 1 CUP | 6 | 160 | 22 | 6 | 17 | 248 | 2.9 |
| TOMATO SOUP W/ WATER, CANNED 1 CUP | 2 | 85 | 17 | 2 | 0 | 244 | 0.4 |
| TOMATO VEG SOUP, DEHYD,PREPRED 1 PKT | 1 | 40 | 8 | 1 | 0 | 189 | 0.3 |
| TOMATOES, CANNED, S+L, W/ SALT 1 CUP | 1 | 50 | 10 | 2 | 0 | 240 | 0.1 |
| TOMATOES, CANNED, S+L,W/O SALT 1 CUP | 1 | 50 | 10 | 2 | 0 | 240 | 0.1 |
| TOMATOES, RAW 1 TOMATO | 0 | 25 | 5 | 1 | 0 | 123 | 0 |
| TORTILLAS, CORN 1 TORTLA | 1 | 65 | 13 | 2 | 0 | 30 | 0.1 |
| TOTAL CEREAL 1 OZ | 1 | 100 | 22 | 3 | 0 | 28.35 | 0.1 |
| TRIX CEREAL 1 OZ | 0 | 110 | 25 | 2 | 0 | 28.35 | 0.2 |
| TROUT, BROILED, W/ BUTTR,LEMJU 3 OZ | 9 | 175 | 0 | 21 | 71 | 85 | 4.1 |
| TUNA SALAD 1 CUP | 19 | 375 | 19 | 33 | 80 | 205 | 3.3 |
| TUNA, CANND, DRND,OIL,CHK,LGHT 3 OZ | 7 | 165 | 0 | 24 | 55 | 85 | 1.4 |
| TUNA, CANND, DRND,WATR, WHITE 3 OZ | 1 | 135 | 0 | 30 | 48 | 85 | 0.3 |
| TURKEY HAM, CURED TURKEY THIGH 2 SLICES | 3 | 75 | 0 | 11 | 32 | 57 | 1 |
| TURKEY LOAF, BREAST MEAT W/O C 2 SLICES | 1 | 45 | 0 | 10 | 17 | 42 | 0.2 |

| Description of food | Fat (Grams) | Food Energy (calories) | Carbohydrate (Grams) | Protein (Grams) | Cholesterol (Milligrams) | Weight (Grams) | Saturated Fat (Grams) |
|---|---|---|---|---|---|---|---|
| TURKEY LOAF, BREAST MEAT, W/ C2 SLICES | 1 | 45 | 0 | 10 | 17 | 42 | 0.2 |
| TURKEY PATTIES, BRD,BATTD,FRID1 PATTY | 12 | 180 | 10 | 9 | 40 | 64 | 3 |
| TURKEY ROAST, FRZN,LGHT+DRK,CK3 OZ | 5 | 130 | 3 | 18 | 45 | 85 | 1.6 |
| TURKEY, ROASTED, DARK MEAT 4 PIECES | 6 | 160 | 0 | 24 | 72 | 85 | 2.1 |
| TURKEY, ROASTED, LIGHT MEAT 2 PIECES | 3 | 135 | 0 | 25 | 59 | 85 | 0.9 |
| TURKEY, ROASTED, LIGHT + DARK 1 CUP | 7 | 240 | 0 | 41 | 106 | 140 | 2.3 |
| TURKEY, ROASTED, LIGHT + DARK 3 PIECES | 4 | 145 | 0 | 25 | 65 | 85 | 1.4 |
| TURNIP GREENS, CKED FRM FROZEN1 CUP | 1 | 50 | 8 | 5 | 0 | 164 | 0.2 |
| TURNIP GREENS, COOKED FROM RAW1 CUP | 0 | 30 | 6 | 2 | 0 | 144 | 0.1 |
| TURNIPS, COOKED, DICED 1 CUP | 0 | 30 | 8 | 1 | 0 | 156 | 0 |
| VANILLA WAFERS 10 COOKE | 7 | 185 | 29 | 2 | 25 | 40 | 1.8 |
| VEAL CUTLET, MED FAT,BRSD,BRLD3 OZ | 9 | 185 | 0 | 23 | 86 | 85 | 4.1 |
| VEAL RIB, MED FAT, ROASTED 3 OZ | 14 | 230 | 0 | 23 | 109 | 85 | 6 |
| VEGETABLE BEEF SOUP, CANNED 1 CUP | 2 | 80 | 10 | 6 | 5 | 244 | 0.9 |
| VEGETABLE JUICE COCKTAIL, CNND1 CUP | 0 | 45 | 11 | 2 | 0 | 242 | 0 |
| VEGETABLES, MIXED, CANNED 1 CUP | 0 | 75 | 15 | 4 | 0 | 163 | 0.1 |
| VEGETABLES, MIXED, CKED FR FRZ1 CUP | 0 | 105 | 24 | 5 | 0 | 182 | 0.1 |
| VEGETARIAN SOUP, CANNED 1 CUP | 2 | 70 | 12 | 2 | 0 | 241 | 0.3 |
| VIENNA BREAD 1 SLICE | 1 | 70 | 13 | 2 | 0 | 25 | 0.2 |
| VIENNA SAUSAGE 1 SAUSAG | 4 | 45 | 0 | 2 | 8 | 16 | 1.5 |
| VINEGAR AND OIL SALAD DRESSING1 TBSP | 8 | 70 | 0 | 0 | 0 | 16 | 1.5 |
| VINEGAR, CIDER 1 TBSP | 0 | 0 | 1 | 0 | 0 | 15 | 0 |
| WAFFLES, FROM HOME RECIPE 1 WAFFLE | 13 | 245 | 26 | 7 | 102 | 75 | 4 |
| WAFFLES, FROM MIX 1 WAFFLE | 8 | 205 | 27 | 7 | 59 | 75 | 2.7 |
| WALNUTS, BLACK, CHOPPED 1 CUP | 71 | 760 | 15 | 30 | 0 | 125 | 4.5 |

| Description of food | | Fat (Grams) | Food Energy (calories) | Carbohydrate (Grams) | Protein (Grams) | Cholesterol (Milligrams) | Weight (Grams) | Saturated Fat (Grams) |
|---|---|---|---|---|---|---|---|---|
| WALNUTS, BLACK, CHOPPED | 1 OZ | 16 | 170 | 3 | 7 | 0 | 28.35 | 1 |
| WALNUTS, ENGLISH, PIECES | 1 CUP | 74 | 770 | 22 | 17 | 0 | 120 | 6.7 |
| WALNUTS, ENGLISH, PIECES | 1 OZ | 18 | 180 | 5 | 4 | 0 | 28.35 | 1.6 |
| WATER CHESTNUTS, CANNED | 1 CUP | 0 | 70 | 17 | 1 | 0 | 140 | 0 |
| WATERMELON, RAW | 1 PIECE | 2 | 155 | 35 | 3 | 0 | 482 | 0.3 |
| WATERMELON, RAW, DICED | 1 CUP | 1 | 50 | 11 | 1 | 0 | 160 | 0.1 |
| WHEAT BREAD | 1 LOAF | 19 | 1160 | 213 | 43 | 0 | 454 | 3.9 |
| WHEAT BREAD | 1 SLICE | 1 | 65 | 12 | 2 | 0 | 25 | 0.2 |
| WHEAT BREAD, TOASTED | 1 SLICE | 1 | 65 | 12 | 3 | 0 | 23 | 0.2 |
| WHEAT FLOUR, ALL-PURPOSE,SIFTD | 1 CUP | 1 | 420 | 88 | 12 | 0 | 115 | 0.2 |
| WHEAT FLOUR, ALL-PURPOSE,UNSIF | 1 CUP | 1 | 455 | 95 | 13 | 0 | 125 | 0.2 |
| WHEATIES CEREAL | 1 OZ | 0 | 100 | 23 | 3 | 0 | 28.35 | 0.1 |
| WHEAT, THIN CRACKERS | 4 CRACKR | 1 | 35 | 5 | 1 | 0 | 8 | 0.5 |
| WHIPPED TOPPING, PRESSURIZED | 1 CUP | 13 | 155 | 7 | 2 | 46 | 60 | 8.3 |
| WHIPPED TOPPING, PRESSURIZED | 1 TBSP | 1 | 10 | 0 | 0 | 2 | 3 | 0.4 |
| WHIPPING CREAM, UNWHIPED,HEAVY | 1 CUP | 88 | 820 | 7 | 5 | 326 | 238 | 54.8 |
| WHIPPING CREAM, UNWHIPED,HEAVY | 1 TBSP | 6 | 50 | 0 | 0 | 21 | 15 | 3.5 |
| WHIPPING CREAM, UNWHIPED,LIGHT | 1 CUP | 74 | 700 | 7 | 5 | 265 | 239 | 46.2 |
| WHIPPING CREAM, UNWHIPED,LIGHT | 1 TBSP | 5 | 45 | 0 | 0 | 17 | 15 | 2.9 |
| WHITE BREAD | 1 LOAF | 18 | 1210 | 222 | 38 | 0 | 454 | 5.6 |
| WHITE BREAD CRUMBS, SOFT | 1 CUP | 2 | 120 | 22 | 4 | 0 | 45 | 0.6 |
| WHITE BREAD CUBES | 1 CUP | 1 | 80 | 15 | 2 | 0 | 30 | 0.4 |
| WHITE BREAD, SLICE 18 PER LOAF | 1 SLICE | 1 | 65 | 12 | 2 | 0 | 25 | 0.3 |
| WHITE BREAD, SLICE 22 PER LOAF | 1 SLICE | 1 | 55 | 10 | 2 | 0 | 20 | 0.2 |
| WHITE BREAD, TOASTED 18 PER | 1 SLICE | 1 | 65 | 12 | 2 | 0 | 22 | 0.3 |

| Description of food | Fat (Grams) | Food Energy (calories) | Carbohydrate (Grams) | Protein (Grams) | Cholesterol (Milligrams) | Weight (Grams) | Saturated Fat (Grams) |
|---|---|---|---|---|---|---|---|
| WHITE BREAD, TOASTED 22 PER 1 SLICE | 1 | 55 | 10 | 2 | 0 | 17 | 0.2 |
| WHITE CAKE W/ WHT FRSTNG,COMML1 CAKE | 148 | 4170 | 670 | 43 | 46 | 1140 | 33.1 |
| WHITE CAKE W/ WHT FRSTNG,COMML1 PIECE | 9 | 260 | 42 | 3 | 3 | 71 | 2.1 |
| WHITE SAUCE W/ MILK FROM MIX 1 CUP | 13 | 240 | 21 | 10 | 34 | 264 | 6.4 |
| WHITE SAUCE, MEDIUM, HOME RECP1 CUP | 30 | 395 | 24 | 10 | 32 | 250 | 9.1 |
| WHOLE-WHEAT BREAD 1 LOAF | 20 | 1110 | 206 | 44 | 0 | 454 | 5.8 |
| WHOLE-WHEAT BREAD 1 SLICE | 1 | 70 | 13 | 3 | 0 | 28 | 0.4 |
| WHOLE-WHEAT BREAD, TOASTED 1 SLICE | 1 | 70 | 13 | 3 | 0 | 25 | 0.4 |
| WHOLE-WHEAT FLOUR,HRD WHT,STIR1 CUP | 2 | 400 | 85 | 16 | 0 | 120 | 0.3 |
| WHOLE-WHEAT WAFERS, CRACKERS 2 CRACKR | 2 | 35 | 5 | 1 | 0 | 8 | 0.5 |
| WINE, DESSERT 3.5 F OZ | 0 | 140 | 8 | 0 | 0 | 103 | 0 |
| WINE, TABLE, RED 3.5 F OZ | 0 | 75 | 3 | 0 | 0 | 102 | 0 |
| WINE, TABLE, WHITE 3.5 F OZ | 0 | 80 | 3 | 0 | 0 | 102 | 0 |
| YEAST, BAKERS, DRY, ACTIVE 1 PKG | 0 | 20 | 3 | 3 | 0 | 7 | 0 |
| YEAST, BREWERS, DRY 1 TBSP | 0 | 25 | 3 | 3 | 0 | 8 | 0 |
| YELLOW CAKE W/ CHOC FRST,FRMIX1 CAKE | 125 | 3735 | 638 | 45 | 576 | 1108 | 47.8 |
| YELLOW CAKE W/ CHOC FRST,FRMIX1 PIECE | 8 | 235 | 40 | 3 | 36 | 69 | 3 |
| YELLOWCAKE W/ CHOCFRSTNG,COMML1 CAKE | 175 | 3895 | 620 | 40 | 609 | 1108 | 92 |
| YELLOWCAKE W/ CHOCFRSTNG,COMML1 PIECE | 11 | 245 | 39 | 2 | 38 | 69 | 5.7 |
| YOGURT, W/ LOFAT MILK, PLAIN 8 OZ | 4 | 145 | 16 | 12 | 14 | 227 | 2.3 |
| YOGURT, W/ LOFAT MILK,FRUITFLV8 OZ | 2 | 230 | 43 | 10 | 10 | 227 | 1.6 |
| YOGURT, W/ NONFAT MILK 8 OZ | 0 | 125 | 17 | 13 | 4 | 227 | 0.3 |
| YOGURT, W/ WHOLE MILK 8 OZ | 7 | 140 | 11 | 8 | 29 | 227 | 4.8 |